S0-AHF-772

HKAC

FEB 2023

Hearing Loss

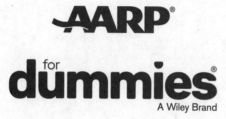

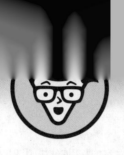

Hearing Loss

by Frank Lin, MD, PhD, and
Nicholas Reed, AuD

AARP®

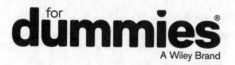
for **dummies**®
A Wiley Brand

Hearing Loss For Dummies®

Published by: **John Wiley & Sons, Inc.**, 111 River Street, Hoboken, NJ 07030-5774, www.wiley.com

Copyright © 2022 by John Wiley & Sons, Inc.

AARP is a registered trademark. All rights reserved.

Any textual or illustrative material prepared for the Work by the Publisher at its expense may be copyrighted separately in the Publisher's name.

Published simultaneously in Canada

No part of this publication may be reproduced, stored in a retrieval system or transmitted in any form or by any means, electronic, mechanical, photocopying, recording, scanning or otherwise, except as permitted under Sections 107 or 108 of the 1976 United States Copyright Act, without the prior written permission of the Publisher. Requests to the Publisher for permission should be addressed to the Permissions Department, John Wiley & Sons, Inc., 111 River Street, Hoboken, NJ 07030, (201) 748-6011, fax (201) 748-6008, or online at http://www.wiley.com/go/permissions.

Trademarks: Wiley, For Dummies, the Dummies Man logo, Dummies.com, Making Everything Easier, and related trade dress are trademarks or registered trademarks of John Wiley & Sons, Inc., and may not be used without written permission. AARP is a registered trademark of AARP, Inc. All other trademarks are the property of their respective owners. John Wiley & Sons, Inc., is not associated with any product or vendor mentioned in this book.

LIMIT OF LIABILITY/DISCLAIMER OF WARRANTY: WHILE THE PUBLISHER, AARP, AND THE AUTHORS HAVE USED THEIR BEST EFFORTS IN PREPARING THIS BOOK, THEY MAKE NO REPRESENTATIONS OR WARRANTIES WITH RESPECT TO THE ACCURACY OR COMPLETENESS OF THE CONTENTS OF THIS BOOK AND SPECIFICALLY DISCLAIM ANY IMPLIED WARRANTIES OF MERCHANTABILITY OR FITNESS FOR A PARTICULAR PURPOSE. NO WARRANTY MAY BE CREATED OR EXTENDED BY SALES REPRESENTATIVES OR WRITTEN SALES MATERIALS. THE ADVICE AND STRATEGIES CONTAINED HEREIN MAY NOT BE SUITABLE FOR YOUR SITUATION. YOU SHOULD CONSULT WITH A PROFESSIONAL WHERE APPROPRIATE. IF PROFESSIONAL ASSISTANCE IS REQUIRED, THE SERVICES OF A COMPETENT PROFESSIONAL PERSON SHOULD BE SOUGHT. THE PUBLISHER, AARP, AND THE AUTHORS SHALL NOT BE LIABLE FOR DAMAGES ARISING HEREFROM. THE FACT THAT AN ORGANIZATION OR WEBSITE IS REFERRED TO IN THIS WORK AS A CITATION AND/OR A POTENTIAL SOURCE OF FURTHER INFORMATION DOES NOT MEAN THAT THE PUBLISHER, AARP, OR THE AUTHORS ENDORSE THE INFORMATION THE ORGANIZATION OR WEBSITE MAY PROVIDE OR RECOMMENDATIONS IT MAY MAKE. FURTHER, READERS SHOULD BE AWARE THAT INTERNET WEBSITES LISTED IN THIS WORK MAY HAVE CHANGED OR DISAPPEARED BETWEEN WHEN THIS WORK WAS WRITTEN AND WHEN IT IS READ.

For general information on our other products and services, please contact our Customer Care Department within the U.S. at 877-762-2974, outside the U.S. at 317-572-3993, or fax 317-572-4002. For technical support, please visit www.wiley.com/techsupport.

Wiley publishes in a variety of print and electronic formats and by print-on-demand. Some material included with standard print versions of this book may not be included in e-books or in print-on-demand. If this book refers to media such as a CD or DVD that is not included in the version you purchased, you may download this material at http://booksupport.wiley.com. For more information about Wiley products, visit www.wiley.com.

Library of Congress Control Number: 2022941589

ISBN 978-1-119-88057-8 (pbk); ISBN 978-1-119-88058-5 (epdf); ISBN 978-1-119-88059-2 (epub)

SKY10035364_071822

Contents at a Glance

Table of Contents

Introduction

You've arrived on the first page of the first edition of *Hearing Loss For Dummies*. When AARP and *For Dummies* asked us to write this book about hearing loss for adults, we jumped with excitement. We, your authors (Frank and Nick), have dedicated our lives to addressing hearing loss [or hearing loss care] through public health research, advocacy for solutions through public policy, and the clinical management of hearing loss. To us, the need was obvious, but perhaps you may be wondering why an entire book is necessary.

Hearing loss among adults is startlingly common. Nearly half of all adults over the age of 60 years have hearing loss. Scientists and clinicians are just now understanding that treating hearing loss is important for our emotional, cognitive, and even physical health. In fact, recent research suggests hearing loss is a risk factor for social isolation, loneliness, falls, cognitive decline, and dementia.

Yet very few people recognize they have hearing loss, and fewer still seek treatment.

In our opinion, the reasons hearing loss is so overlooked and hearing care neglected include these:

>> Hearing loss sets in so slowly and subtly over time that many people don't even realize what they're missing.

>> Society has painted hearing loss as an inconsequential aspect of aging with, until recently, little understanding of how it impacts our overall health.

>> Hearing care, such as hearing aids, can be a costly and timely endeavor that isn't covered by most insurance, including Medicare.

>> Hearing aids get a bad rap. People think it's a sign of aging, when in reality, addressing hearing loss keeps you vibrant and engaged.

>> Hearing loss is complex and confusing. For example: What's mild hearing loss, and is it important? What's a high-frequency or low-frequency hearing loss? What do all those graphs and numbers from a hearing test mean? What hearing aids and other treatments are available?

But so much has changed in just the past decade or so that the time is now right for this book.

Given the explosion of research on the importance of addressing hearing loss, Congress has approved a new category of more affordable over-the-counter hearing aids intended for sale directly to adults without the need for a professional. At press time, these new hearing aids, aimed at people with mild to moderate hearing loss, are slated to be available in late 2022. In addition, new public health initiatives have emerged to move away from vague terminology and graphs when explaining hearing loss to simple and actionable numbers that are easier for people to grasp and more clearly show how hearing changes over time.

That's a lot of change in a short time period, and *Hearing Loss For Dummies* is here to break it all down for you and provide a road map for your hearing health journey.

About This Book

If you're feeling overwhelmed with where to start in understanding how hearing loss happens and what can be done about it, you've come to the right place. This book is intended to act as an easy-to-read reference guide, giving you practical knowledge and actionable solutions to address hearing loss and how it affects your everyday life.

This book focuses on hearing loss in adults that develops over time. (We do not cover the complex nature of hearing loss in children, nor do we go into rare and complex medically related hearing loss in adults.) Simply put, the inner ear was not made to last forever. Every single person on this planet experiences a decline in hearing ability as they age, and most over a certain age (around 60) develop a level of hearing loss that is sufficient to begin interfering with their daily lives and is linked with an increased risk of poorer health, falls, social isolation, cognitive decline, and dementia.

To help you navigate what occurs with hearing loss, we cover risk factors for hearing loss and touch on types of hearing loss for adults. We also walk you through the process of taking a hearing test and reading your results as well as give helpful information on purchasing hearing aids — either prescription hearing aids through a professional or over-the-counter hearing aids — and seeking support as you manage your hearing loss.

Foolish Assumptions

This book assumes you know nothing about and have no prior knowledge of hearing loss. Nothing. Nada. Zero. We explain terms and concepts in plain language. But even if you already know a lot about hearing loss, we think you'll find this book helpful as we take some deeper dives into concepts and offer practical advice from years of clinical care and research.

If you find yourself answering "yes" to any of the following, you'll find information in this book for you:

>> Do you suspect you have hearing loss but don't know where to start?

>> Have you heard about the new (at the time of this book) category of over-the-counter hearing aids and want information to make an informed decision on your purchase?

>> Do you have a loved one or friend with hearing loss and want to support them?

>> Are you new to hearing aids, and do you want a reference book with practical tips and tricks for using them?

>> Have you recently learned you have hearing loss and are looking for a guide to your options in hearing care?

>> Do you think you may need hearing aids but are reluctant to start the process?

>> Do you just want to know more about hearing loss?

Icons Used in This Book

You'll see various icons throughout this book. They're meant to complement the material and are our way of pointing out what is essential information versus what is nice to know but can be skipped without affecting your ability to get the right message. Here's what each icon means:

REMEMBER

This icon refers to fundamental and important information on hearing loss that shouldn't be ignored.

WARNING

This icon raises awareness of potential misunderstandings or easy-to-make mistakes in hearing care such as avoiding certain predatory situations in purchasing a hearing aid.

TIP

This icon marks important and practical advice and insights.

TECHNICAL STUFF

If you see this icon, it means that what follows is probably just your authors giving you scientific details you don't absolutely need but we find super interesting. Feel free to ignore information with this icon without sacrificing take-home knowledge.

Beyond the Book

In addition to the content in this book, we've created online Cheat Sheets for quick access to important information in this book, including hearing loss basics, guidelines for testing and care, communication tips, and major Dos and Don'ts of hearing aids. The Cheat Sheets can be found at www.dummies.com by typing "Hearing Loss For Dummies Cheat Sheet" in the Search bar.

Where to Go from Here

This book was never intended to be read cover to cover. Don't get us wrong; feel free to do so if you are inclined, but you won't hurt our feelings if you don't.

We wrote this book as a reference guide using plain language and plenty of examples to present advanced concepts. The book is designed for each chapter to stand alone so you can jump in at any place to find information you need at that moment. We also understand that sometimes reading one section can create new questions, so we regularly point you to other places in the book for related topics. Of course, you're always free to check out the table of contents or the index. Start wherever suits your needs. For example:

>> Need a broad overview of everything? Start with Chapter 1.

>> Concerned you may have hearing loss? Skip to Chapter 5 for some signs of hearing loss.

>> You already know the basics of hearing loss, have already had a hearing test, and now are thinking about hearing treatment? Start with Chapters 8 and 9.

>> Want some tips on hearing better at work, at home, in social settings, and in public places? Turn to Chapter 12.

>> Want to find out more about whether you're a good fit for the new over-the-counter hearing aids? Check out Chapter 10.

>> Want some help navigating insurance and government benefits related to hearing loss? Jump to Chapters 15 and 16.

>> You bought this book because a friend or loved one has hearing loss and you want to find out how to support them? Chapter 14 is for you.

1
Understanding Hearing Loss

Learn how hearing naturally declines over time and why it matters to recognize hearing loss and the role it plays in everyday life.

Uncover how the ear and brain work together to recognize sound.

Review causes of hearing loss.

Discover the link between your hearing and your health and well-being.

Chapter **1**

Cheers to Your Ears!

heers, indeed! It's not often that we take a moment to appreciate what our ears — and more importantly our ability to hear — allow us to do!

From the clink of two wine glasses coming gently together to the word "Cheers" itself, your ability to hear allows you to process and understand the world around you. Enjoying a conversation over dinner, appreciating the melody and voices of a choir, pulling to the side of the road at the sound of a fire engine . . . it's all made possible by your hearing!

For all of us, though, our hearing will gradually and subtly decline over time. By the time we're in our 40s, 7% of us will experience some hearing loss. By our 60s, that number grows to 27%, and by our 80s and older, 82%. Hearing loss is inevitable even for those of us who didn't attend loud concerts or crank up the volume in our earbuds. Yet all too often, people perceive hearing loss as a relatively inconsequential aspect of aging.

Scientists now know that nothing could be further from the truth. Addressing hearing loss may be one of the most important things you can do to keep your body and brain healthy and to keep you engaged with life. This chapter takes you on a tour of why we all develop hearing loss, why it matters, and most importantly, what you can — and should — do about it. Hearing loss isn't about growing old. Rather, addressing hearing loss is one thing we can do to keep us engaged with our families, friends, and colleagues in our everyday lives. This book is all about understanding hearing loss, what you can do about it, and the joys and benefits to health and well-being that hearing brings to your daily life.

Understanding Why Hearing Loss Happens

Knowledge is power! If you're reading this book, you may be concerned about what you should know about hearing loss and what can be done about it. This chapter gives you an overview of the information you need to understand what's happening and the steps you can take to hear better.

Hearing takes place over two steps

The sounds we hear every day — like someone's voice, a piece of music, or a fire engine — are complex and made up of a mosaic of thousands of individual sounds of different pitches and intensities. The first step in being able to hear is that your inner ear (the *cochlea*) converts this mishmash of different sounds with perfect precision into a signal that is transmitted to the brain. (For more on how your ears and hearing work, turn to Chapter 2.)

Imagine recording a symphony with a fancy microphone and a computer. The microphone picks up the complicated, rich music in the symphony hall and encodes it into a stream of data that can be analyzed and recorded on the computer. Your cochlea is basically doing the same thing as the microphone in picking up the sounds that come to your ear and encoding these sounds into electrical signals (data) that are transmitted to your brain.

The second step of hearing occurs when your brain receives the signal (or "data") from the ear and decodes it into meaning. Your brain can nearly instantaneously decode the signal into whether the sound you just heard was someone saying your name, a melody in your favorite piece of music, the fire engine roaring down the street, or perhaps all three at the same time! To do this, your brain relies not only on the data sent from your ear but also additional cues as well. For example, when decoding speech sounds, your brain also relies on knowing the context of the conversation and seeing the movements of the speaker's lips.

Hearing loss happens as the inner ear wears out

There are many different types of and causes of hearing loss, but in this book, we're covering the most common type of hearing loss that all of us will develop to some degree over time. This type of *sensorineural* hearing loss (see Chapter 2) develops over time as parts of the inner ear wear out gradually. The inner ear is made up of highly specialized cells responsible for converting sounds into a neural signal. Unfortunately, unlike other cells in the body, these specialized cells of the inner ear (called sensory hair cells) can't regenerate once they wear out and have become damaged. In contrast, cells in other parts of your body, like your brain, liver, and heart, can all gradually be replaced over time by new cells.

As these cells of the inner ear wear out over time and are lost, the inner ear becomes less effective at accurately encoding the sounds entering your ear into a precise neural signal. In this case, your brain still receives data from the ear, but instead of being crystal clear, the data comes across as garbled and unclear. That's why for anyone with hearing loss, it sounds as if other people aren't speaking clearly or are mumbling. You may not even notice that your hearing is getting worse over time, because it can happen very gradually and subtly. Certain sounds may just sound a little fuzzy or garbled, but you may not realize it's due to hearing loss.

Factors that affect your hearing over time

Lots of different factors can affect your hearing over time (we detail these in greater depth in Chapter 3), and they can generally be divided into those that are non-modifiable (those you can't control) versus those that are modifiable (ones you *can* control).

Here are some key non-modifiable risk factors:

» **Age:** This is the strongest risk factor for hearing loss. The cells in your ears responsible for hearing degrade over time.

» **Sex:** Compared to men, women in general have better hearing. This may be related to women having increased estrogen that scientists think could protect the inner ear. Women may also have less exposure on average to loud sounds than men.

» **Skin color:** Individuals with darker skin on average are at a lower risk of hearing loss. The amount of melanin in your skin determines your skin color (the more melanin you have, the darker your skin color is), and there's a corresponding amount of melanin in your inner ear. Scientists believe this inner ear melanin helps protect the inner ear over time.

The most important modifiable risk factors for hearing loss include these:

» **Noise:** This is by far the most important risk factor you can control. As a general rule of thumb, if you're in an environment or situation where you consistently have to raise your voice to be heard, you should move away from the noise if you can or consider using some form of ear protection such as earplugs or over-the-ear noise-canceling headphones or earmuffs. You'll also want to avoid listening to music through headphones or earbuds for too long or too loud. See Chapter 3 for tips on how to use headphones safely and information on how noise affects hearing.

» **Cardiovascular risk factors:** There are myriad risk factors for cardiovascular disease such as smoking, hypertension, and diabetes, and all these can also increase your risk for hearing loss by damaging the small blood vessels that go to your ear. Head to Chapter 3 for more information.

Putting Hearing Loss in Context

Everyone loses some hearing with age. What we want to stress is just how common it is; how it can impact your physical, emotional, and cognitive health; and what you can do to hear better.

Hearing loss happens to everyone

If you're concerned about hearing loss, you are most certainly not alone!

The number of people who experience hearing loss is staggering, as Figure 1-1 shows.

In this figure you can see that the percentage of people with hearing loss nearly doubles with every decade of aging. The figure also gives an indication of the relative severity of the hearing loss divided into those with mild and moderate or worse hearing loss. These concepts are covered in more detail in Chapter 7.

How hearing loss impacts our health and well-being

Scientists didn't always understand much about the consequences of hearing loss for adults. The general impression among even doctors was that since everyone developed some hearing problems over time, it couldn't possibly be that bad for health.

That period has now passed.

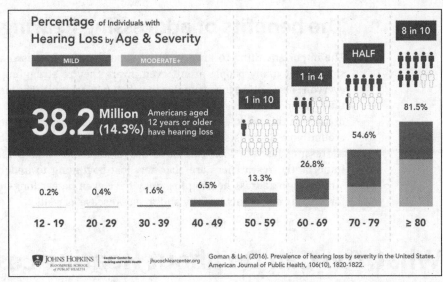

FIGURE 1-1:
Prevalence of
hearing loss in
the United States.

Source: Johns Hopkins Cochlear Center for Hearing and Public Health

Research over the past decade has increasingly demonstrated the adverse effects that hearing loss can have on our health. Key areas where scientists now believe that hearing loss increases our risk for adverse health events include cognitive, emotional, social, and physical areas of health:

>> **Cognitive impairment and dementia:** Research suggests that of all the known treatable risk factors for dementia, hearing loss may be the single largest contributor to dementia risk. Scientists think this is because hearing loss makes it harder for our brain to process sound, and individuals with hearing loss are less likely to remain engaged in social and other stimulating activities that are critical to cognitive health.

>> **Loneliness:** Feeling withdrawn and detached from others is strongly linked with poor health outcomes like early mortality, heart attacks, and cognitive decline. Hearing loss contributes to loneliness because it makes it harder for people to socially engage with others.

>> **Falls:** Hearing is one of several systems — including our vision, *vestibular* (balance), cardiovascular, pulmonary, and *proprioception* (sense of touch) systems — that allow our brain to maintain our body's balance.

Importantly, while scientists now understand that hearing loss likely contributes meaningfully to all these adverse outcomes, they don't know yet whether our current treatments for hearing loss (for example, using hearing aids) may lower this risk. Studies are ongoing, and scientists are hopeful.

The benefits of addressing hearing loss

The important thing to keep in mind about hearing loss is that it comes on so slowly that many people aren't even aware they're struggling to hear (despite everyone else noting the struggles the person is having!). The single most important reason to address your hearing loss — with the strategies and technologies detailed in this book — is so that you can fully engage with others and the world around you. Scientists and doctors have long known the positive benefits that addressing hearing loss can have on relationships and personal well-being. Importantly, researchers are also now just beginning to understand that these strategies to address hearing loss may have even bigger long-term implications for keeping our brains healthy and free of disease as well!

What You Can Do about Hearing Loss

Besides avoiding loud noises and protecting cardiovascular health, what can you do about hearing loss? It can't be cured, but it most certainly can be addressed with a range of strategies to allow individuals with hearing loss to communicate and hear optimally. When it comes to hearing loss and how it affects you, you are the master of your own destiny. You don't have to sit back and just let hearing loss adversely impact your life. There are strategies and technologies to combat these effects so you can remain fully engaged with the richness of the world around you (see Chapters 8 through 13 for details on these).

Know your hearing

This may seem obvious, but to address hearing loss, you first need to know whether in fact you have hearing loss! In many cases, as you can tell from Figure 1-1, you may have a pretty good idea already based purely on your age (nearly two-thirds of everyone over 70 has hearing loss) and the symptoms you may be experiencing. Subjective impressions of your hearing can be helpful, but in most cases, you'll be far better informed if you have an objective hearing test.

Get your hearing checked

Hearing tests are most commonly performed by an audiologist or a hearing instrument specialist. Ideally, you want to start with an audiologist since these are health professionals trained to diagnose and treat hearing loss, and health insurance will nearly always cover the exam. Depending on your insurance, you may need a medical referral. An audiologist can perform a comprehensive hearing exam and then discuss your evaluation and possible options to address any hearing or communication problems you may be experiencing.

Hearing instrument specialists can also assess your hearing. They are licensed by the state to sell hearing aids and to conduct hearing tests expressly for the purposes of possibly fitting a hearing aid. Hearing instrument specialists often offer these hearing tests for free, but their ultimate hope is that you'll then buy a hearing aid from them. There's nothing wrong with these tests, but just be forewarned that they may also come with a sales pitch.

You may also want to consider having your hearing evaluated by an ear, nose, and throat (ENT) physician (also called an *otolaryngologist*), particularly if you have any medical concerns about your hearing. An ENT is trained in the medical and surgical management of hearing loss and often works with an audiologist in the office. The audiologist performs the hearing evaluation, and the ENT then examines your ears and evaluates whether you have any medically or surgically treatable issues related to your hearing loss. Consult an ENT if you notice any of the following:

>> Drainage from your ears

>> Ear pain

>> Asymmetrical hearing between your ears

>> Sudden or fluctuating hearing loss (see an ENT immediately if your hearing loss comes on suddenly)

>> Dizziness or vertigo

>> Hearing loss that has not been significantly helped by using hearing aids in the past

Turn to Chapter 6 for a full rundown on hearing professionals and tests.

Get your hearing number

One of the best ways to get a better grasp and understanding of your hearing is to know your hearing number. The hearing number — known clinically as the speech-frequency pure-tone average — indicates how loud on average speech sounds have to be for you to hear them. The larger your hearing number, the worse your hearing is.

You will get this number from your hearing test. You can also calculate it from a hearing test yourself using your own smartphone (see Chapter 7).

You can find more details about the hearing number — how it's calculated and what it means — in Chapter 7 and at www.hearingnumber.org, part of an effort by the Johns Hopkins Bloomberg School of Public Health, where both authors are based, to increase public awareness and knowledge around hearing loss.

In general, the greater your hearing number is, the more communication strategies and technologies you'll want to consider using to allow you to hear and communicate optimally.

Using communication strategies

The most important way for you or a loved one to optimize hearing and communication is with some basic communication strategies. These strategies can help with communication because they focus on getting a clearer sound to your ear.

"How does this help with hearing?" you may ask. The cells in the inner ear break down over time, as we mention earlier in the chapter, and the inner ear can no longer convert sound into the signal that goes to the brain as accurately as it once did. As a result, the signal that reaches the brain sounds garbled or fuzzy; you may complain that people are mumbling.

In a situation where the incoming sound was very clear to begin with, some slight garbling in the encoding process in the inner can still lead to a fairly clear signal reaching the brain that is easily understandable. In contrast, say the incoming sound was already fuzzy to begin with (imagine trying to hear someone over the din of a loud cocktail party). The inner ear with hearing loss then further garbles the sound during the encoding process, and the resulting signal to the brain may be completely unintelligible.

The communication strategies summarized here and covered in greater depth in Chapter 8 can enhance the quality of the incoming sound and/or provide the listener with additional cues to help their brain understand sound. Important communication strategies to keep in mind are

>> Get close to (within arm's length) and face-to-face with people you're talking to.

>> Turn down or move away from any background noise whenever possible when talking to others.

>> At restaurants or other indoor places, choose rooms that are smaller and have lower ceilings and lots of soft surfaces (such as curtains and rugs), which reduce the amount of reverberation that can markedly degrade sound quality.

>> Instead of saying "Huh?" or "What?" when you can't understand what someone has said, be specific about what you did and didn't hear. For example, "I heard you say something about meeting for dinner but missed the rest." This takes a bit longer but cues the speaker into exactly what to repeat and shows that you were listening (so you aren't accused by your spouse of never paying attention!).

Hearing technologies

Yes, technology can indeed be a huge help when it comes to optimizing your ability to hear and communicate with hearing loss. But the *most important* thing is to manage your expectations. Hearing technology — such as hearing aids and cochlear implants — can improve your hearing, but no matter how much you pay, it can never completely fix your damaged inner ear and its degraded ability to accurately encode sounds.

That being said, when these technologies — such as hearing aids and cochlear implants — are appropriately used and programmed for your hearing loss, they can make a *huge* life-changing difference in your ability to navigate your day with ease. Keep in mind, though, that when using such technologies, the benefits aren't always noticeable immediately. It often takes a few months for your brain to get used to and benefit from the new sounds that a hearing aid or cochlear implant provides. Think of using a new set of hearing aids like learning to ride a bike for the first time. You may not like it at first, but over time as your brain gets used to the sounds from the hearing aids and learns how to use them, the benefits can be remarkable.

Hearing aids

Hearing aids are the foundational technology for many people with hearing loss, and prescription hearing aids are typically purchased through a hearing care professional who will provide you with support services to ensure you're able to benefit from the hearing aids. This model of hearing care delivery where you have to get your hearing aids through a hearing care provider works well for some people but is not necessarily ideal for everyone.

A new and exciting development is happening, though, as this book goes to press in 2022. Beginning in late 2022, hearing aids in the United States will soon be available not just as prescription but also as over-the-counter (OTC) devices.

OTC hearing aid regulations at the time of publication are just being finalized by the U.S. Food and Drug Administration (FDA). Once these regulations are enacted in late 2022, manufacturers will be able to develop and sell OTC hearing aids that meet specific acoustic performance criteria to ensure that these hearing aids are both safe and effective for consumers without the need for an audiologist or hearing instrument specialist. These OTC hearing aids will be specifically for adults with mild to moderate levels of hearing loss, which is what the vast majority — over 90 percent — of people with hearing loss have. (When purchasing OTC hearing aids, you may still want to consult with a professional to best understand which devices to consider and how to best use them.)

In contrast, prescription hearing aids will still continue to be available through an audiologist or hearing instrument specialist. People who have greater severity levels of hearing loss, who have other ear or audiological issues, and who need a much more customized hearing aid because of their listening needs will still need prescription devices.

Thriving with hearing aids means setting appropriate expectations for what hearing aids can and can't do (hint: they don't restore hearing to normal), practicing with your hearing aids to get used to them, and creating good care and maintenance routines. Your actions can make all the difference in whether or not you succeed with hearing aids. Understanding this is especially important when pursuing OTC hearing aids without the guidance and input of a professional.

To get more information and answers to your hearing aid questions and tips for thriving with hearing aids, check out Chapters 9 through 12.

Cochlear implants

Cochlear implants are indicated for adults who have hearing loss in the severe range and no longer find adequate benefit from using a hearing aid. A cochlear implant is a surgically implanted *neuroprothesis* that converts sounds into electrical signals that are then directly sent by the cochlear implant to the brain via the hearing nerve (see Chapter 13 for more information). In this way, the cochlear implant takes the place of the cochlea, and thus, is a prosthesis.

Cochlear implants have been around for more than 30 years and are a routine outpatient day surgery for any ENT who specializes in ear surgeries. (Nearly all academic medical centers and large private-practice ENT groups offer this surgery.)

As a general rule of thumb, if you or a loved one still struggle with communication despite using hearing aids and have a moderately severe or greater hearing loss (with a hearing number somewhere in the 60s or worse — see Chapter 7), you may want to consider being evaluated to see if you're a candidate for a cochlear implant. This evaluation is routinely covered by insurance and is generally offered by any academic medical center or larger private-practice ENT group.

In the past, the FDA approved cochlear implants only for individuals with severe hearing loss in both ears. Recently, that changed. Cochlear implants are also now indicated for individuals with severe or greater hearing loss in just one ear (also called single-sided deafness, or SSD). Not all insurance plans, though, cover a cochlear implant for SSD.

Getting the Support You Need

Addressing hearing loss may at times may seem like it's solely the responsibility of the person with hearing loss, but nothing could be further from the truth! When a person struggles with communication, it's as much the individual's concern as well as the other people they're trying to speak with.

Surprisingly, most people never learn what to do to help others with hearing problems despite the vast number of people with hearing loss. Chapter 14 explains how a person's hearing loss can have cascading effects on others and the various strategies that can allow people to support them. Options for covering hearing care either through insurance or out-of-pocket (Chapter 15) and a person's legal rights under the Americans with Disabilities Act and other federal policies (Chapter 16) pertaining to hearing loss are also covered in Part 4 of the book.

Chapter **2**

Understanding How Hearing Works

Every day, everywhere, and at any time, you're surrounded by sounds that you may not even be consciously aware of — the hum of the refrigerator in a seemingly quiet kitchen, your footsteps hitting the ground on a walk, or the rustle of the sheets as you shift in bed. These sounds are layered onto the ones that may be more obvious, such as a family member's voice or music from the radio. All these sounds combine to keep you in touch with your surroundings.

If your ability to hear certain sounds begins to disappear, the world becomes a different place. Sounds are used to cue you in to your environment and allow you to communicate. If these sounds become distorted or fade away, the way you perceive and interpret things changes.

In this chapter, we show you how your hearing works and why being able to hear and communicate effectively is critical to your health. This knowledge will ultimately empower you to best address any hearing challenges you and others you care about may be facing.

What Is Sound?

At its simplest, sound is just the vibration of air molecules hitting one another all around you and creating sound waves that move through the air. Consider the sound of a piano: A felt-covered wooden hammer strikes a metal string, which then vibrates the surrounding air. Likewise, the sound of a fork dropped on the kitchen floor comes from the vibrations in the air created by both the fork and the ceramic tile it hits. Similarly, your friend's voice is created when the air exhaled by the lungs passes through the vocal cords in the throat.

Why is this important, you may ask? Well, if you're having trouble hearing, you need to first understand what it is that your ear is indeed trying to hear. Namely, understanding what makes up sounds will let you have a better idea of what your ear is trying to do and why the hearing devices and strategies that we discuss later in this book can help.

How sound gets its sound

Two factors define a sound:

>> **Frequency of the vibrations:** How fast the air molecules vibrate gives sound its pitch — the more rapid the vibrations, the higher the pitch (or frequency) of the sound.

>> **Intensity of the vibrations:** How hard the air molecules hit each other gives sound its loudness — the greater the strength of the collisions, the louder the sound.

The frequency of a sound is indicated by hertz (abbreviated as Hz), where one hertz indicates one vibration per second. Humans can hear sounds ranging from 20 Hz to 15,000–20,000 Hz. (In contrast, a dog's hearing extends from ~60 Hz to 45,000 Hz.)

For perspective about what these frequencies sound like, the lowest note on a standard 88-key piano is about 30 Hz while the highest note is about 4,000 Hz. Sounds in the 10,000–15,000 Hz range are like the brilliant sounds that a cymbal produces.

TECHNICAL
STUFF

The intensity or loudness of a sound is measured in decibels (abbreviated dB), which is a unit of sound pressure. The greater the pressure, the greater the intensity and hence the loudness of the sound. Sounds that we commonly encounter in daily life range generally from 0 dB (barely audible to someone with great hearing) to 120 dB (an ambulance siren up close). In general, every 10 dB increase in a sound's intensity will be perceived as being twice as loud. For example, a 30 dB whisper will be perceived as being twice as loud as a 20 dB soft whisper.

We cover sound frequency and intensity again later in this book, particularly in Chapter 7 as we go over how hearing tests work, so you'll get a better sense then of what these terms and numbers mean to you. The important thing to know now is that all the sounds you hear around you are made up of a smorgasbord of vibrating air molecules, all with different frequencies and intensities that change with every passing second!

What sound "looks" like

We've always liked the adage "A picture is worth a thousand words," so here's our attempt at it.

Figure 2-1 depicts a spectrogram — or visual representation — of the vibrations that make up ten seconds of a Bach piano concerto. The music is made up of a whole slew of different sounds that consist of different frequencies (indicated by the frequency axis) as well as different intensities (indicated by the height of the peaks), and these sounds all progress second by second.

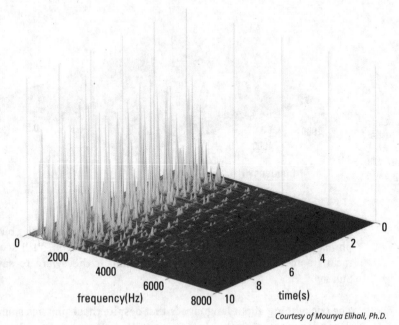

FIGURE 2-1: Visual spectrogram of ten seconds of a Bach piano concerto.

Courtesy of Mounya Elihali, Ph.D.

You can also tell that there's a slightly rhythmic pattern to the spectrogram with many of the peaks of sound coming at regular time intervals. This may not come as a surprise because, well, music has rhythm.

Virtually anything you hear in everyday life can be visualized like this figure — that is, a range of vibrations of different frequencies and intensity that characterize what you hear.

As another example, Figure 2-2 shows the spectrogram for the spoken phrase, "I'll see you Sunday." Most speech sounds that we hear on an everyday basis are primarily clustered between 500 Hz and 4,000 Hz (see more in Chapter 7), and you can see how a snippet of speech looks different from the vibrations of sound that characterize the classical music segment in Figure 2-1.

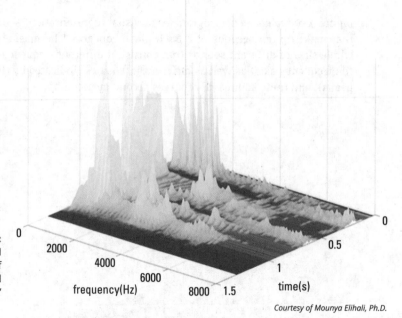

FIGURE 2-2:
Visual spectrogram of the phrase, "I'll see you Sunday."

0   2000   4000   6000   8000   1.5
frequency(Hz)

0   0.5   1   1.5
time(s)

Courtesy of Mounya Elihali, Ph.D.

As a final example, consider Figure 2-3, which depicts a similar but quite different phrase: "I'll see you someday." A friend saying to you, "I'll see you someday" means something completely different than if they were to say, "I'll see you Sunday."

The tricky thing about language is that despite these phrases sounding very similar and, not surprisingly, the spectrograms in Figures 2-2 and 2-3 looking nearly identical, the meaning is completely different — with serious implications for what you'll be doing this upcoming weekend!

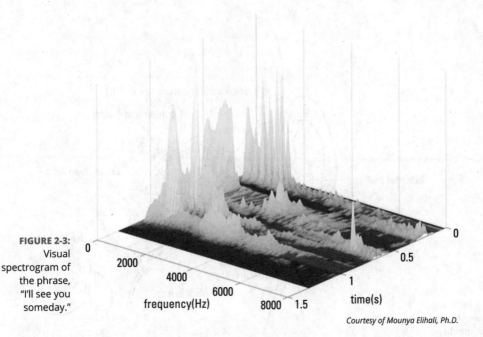

FIGURE 2-3:
Visual spectrogram of the phrase, "I'll see you someday."

0

2000

4000

6000

8000   1.5

frequency(Hz)

0

0.5

1

time(s)

0

Courtesy of Mounya Elihali, Ph.D.

To Hear, You Need Your Ear!

This may be fairly obvious, but the first step in your ability to hear sounds — whether a Bach piano concerto or a friend's passing phrase — involves the ear. While many people think of the ear as being just the part that protrudes from the side of your head, there are actually three parts that make up the ear or what's also called the *peripheral auditory system* (Figure 2-4):

>> **External ear:** Includes the *pinna* (the technical name for the part of the ear that protrudes from the side of your head) and the ear canal that leads to the eardrum (also called the *tympanic membrane*)

>> **Middle ear:** Includes the eardrum and the three ear bones (*ossicles*) that connect the eardrum to the inner ear

>> **Inner ear:** Includes the *cochlea* (a very thin tube about 3 centimeters coiled up into a snail-shaped organ encased in the hardest bone in the body) as well as the semicircular balance canals (also called the *vestibular system*)

The following sections explain what each part of the ear does in more detail. Understanding the basic setup of the ear will help you discover where your or your loved one's hearing problems may be coming from.

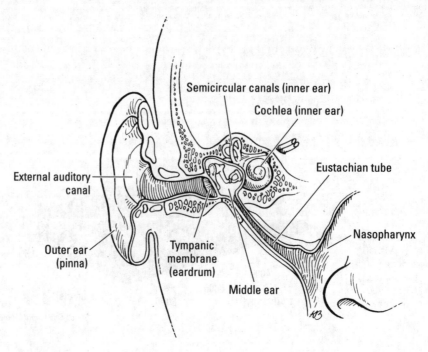

FIGURE 2-4:
Diagram of the
external, middle,
and inner ear.

The labels in the figure read:

Semicircular canals (inner ear)

Cochlea (inner ear)

Eustachian tube

External auditory canal

Nasopharynx

Outer ear (pinna)

Tympanic membrane (eardrum)

Middle ear

External ear

The external ear consists of the pinna and ear canal. The pinna is responsible for collecting the sound waves created by vibrating air molecules and channeling these down the ear canal toward the eardrum. The funnel-shaped design of the pinna and ear canal helps collect and amplify the sounds that are channeled into the middle ear (much like the "ear horns" that people with hearing loss used centuries ago to help amplify sound). The ear canal is also where you get ear wax (cerumen; more on this in Chapter 3) and external ear infections. These infections are often related to water exposure and too much moisture in the ear canal (more on both of these later in this chapter and in Chapter 3).

Middle ear

The middle ear is made up of the eardrum and the three ear bones that connect the eardrum to the inner ear. The main function of the middle ear is to convert the sound waves created by vibrating air molecules into a form of mechanical energy that can be transmitted to the inner ear. The middle ear is filled with air and is connected by the *Eustachian tube*, through which air gets in and out of the middle ear space, to the back of the nose.

Here's how the middle ear works: Sound waves hit and vibrate the eardrum, which in turn leads to the bones of the middle ear moving back and forth. The first ear bone — the *malleus*, attached to the eardrum — moves back and forth as the eardrum vibrates. The malleus in turn rocks the next ear bone, the *incus*, which then moves the last ear bone, the *stapes*, which pushes on the fluid contained in the inner ear.

The system is ingenious in that the middle ear, much like the external ear, also helps amplify the sounds transmitted eventually to the inner ear. This happens because of the physics of sound. Sound vibrations are collected by the eardrum, amplified through a mechanical leverage effect of the three ear bones, and then concentrated into the pressure exerted onto a much smaller area as the stapes pushes into the inner ear.

Inner ear

The cochlea of the inner ear is where the magic happens! Up until this point, the stuff that occurs in the external and middle ear consists basically of the physical effects of sound vibrations being concentrated and converted into the mechanical energy of the moving ear bones. In the cochlea, this mechanical energy (which used to be the energy of vibrating air molecules) gets encoded into an electrical signal that is transmitted via nerve fibers to the brain.

This process happens because the cochlea contains highly specialized hair-like cells that allow the complicated moonscape of sound vibrations, depicted in Figures 2-1 to 2-3, to be converted with perfect fidelity into electrical signals that get sent to the brain. These cells line the length of the coiled-up tube that makes up the cochlea like the keys of a piano. These cells aren't hair per se, like that on top of our head, but they do have microscopic "hairs," called *cilia*, that stick out from the cell.

Scientists have been studying how this process works for decades, and it's complex. The quick summary goes like this:

>> The stapes (the last ear bone) pushes the fluid in the inner ear at one end of the cochlear tube creating waves in the fluid (imagine the rippling waves created when a child jumps into a pool).

>> The waves created by low-frequency sounds (vibrations) travel farther down the length of the tube than the waves created by high-frequency sounds.

>> The waves stimulate sensory hair cells, which trigger an electrical signal via the hearing nerve to the brain.

WHY DO MY EARS FEEL LIKE THEY NEED TO POP?

You likely have encountered at some point in your life having a sense of fullness in your ears that's relieved after you swallow or yawn. You may notice this when you're driving down a mountain or flying in a plane, with the change of air pressure. You feel your ear pop, and it suddenly feels better. What's going on here?

Well, this happens because the opening of the Eustachian tube at the back of the nose has only a narrow, slit-like opening that normally is in a closed position. When you swallow or yawn, muscles in the back of your nose stretch the opening of the Eustachian tube open for just a brief moment, and in this moment, air can go back and forth through the Eustachian tube.

The pressure you felt initially was likely from a mismatch of the air pressure in your middle ear (the air here is constantly getting absorbed by the middle ear lining) and the air pressure in the environment. When you swallow or yawn, air is able to rush back and forth to equalize the pressure, and voilà, the pressure is relieved!

The result of the combined effects of the external, middle, and particularly the inner ear is that sounds that were previously just a mishmash of vibrations of air molecules are converted and encoded with near-perfect fidelity into a series of electrical signals that go to the brain. These electrical signals directly encode and represent the complicated pattern of sound vibrations seen in Figures 2-1 to 2-3.

But amazingly, this is only half the story. What happens next is even more fascinating.

Hearing with Your Brain

You may be surprised to learn how important the brain is for hearing. The process in your ear — a series of electrical signals that encodes sound — seems pretty cool, but how does that allow you to understand what your friend is saying to you across the dinner table? For that, you need your brain! Stated another way, your ear *encodes* sounds into an electrical signal, but your brain then has to *decode* the signal into actual meaning.

Multiple parts of the brain are involved in decoding the signal from the ear, and this primarily happens in portions of the brain's *temporal lobe* (the part of the brain on either side of your head that sits above the ears). We often take this brain processing for granted, but it's pretty amazing that it's so effortless and happens in real time.

Case in point: Even with all the advances in voice recognition technology that we see nowadays (such as Amazon Alexa, Apple Siri, and Google Assistant), these systems still make errors all the time and can't compare to the accuracy of even a young child when it comes to understanding speech.

The following sections reveal how your brain takes signals from both your ears — as well as your other senses and the environment — and converts them into actual meaning.

Two ears are better than one

Your brain is fortunate in that it gets not just one but two auditory signals — from your left and right ears — to help it understand what it's hearing. We refer to the concept of the brain using two signals as *binaural hearing*.

Improving clarity and focus

These two signals are similar but slightly different because the sound that reaches each ear is not the same. For instance, if you're sitting and talking with a friend in a noisy coffee shop, your friend's voice will arrive at each ear a bit differently depending on where they're sitting relative to you. If your friend is sitting a bit closer to your left side, their voice will arrive just a bit sooner and a bit louder in your left ear than your right ear. Amazingly, in processing these sound signals, the brain can use these subtle differences in the two signals to cancel out the background noise and instead focus on the voice you're trying to hear.

Reducing effort and enhancing comfort

Two signals also mean less work for your brain in detecting and deciphering sound. The brain adds up the two signals, which means it can detect softer sounds with two ears better than one. So, with two ears you don't need sound to be as loud, and you can hear sounds from a further distance. In fact, a voice heard from 10 feet away with one ear could be heard from as far as 30 to 40 feet away with two ears! This combining of signals makes listening less effortful and more comfortable.

TIP

The advantage of having both signals is pretty easy to experience. Next time you're in a challenging listening condition (such as trying to understand a speaker in a crowded or noisy room), try listening with one ear covered. You may notice that your brain has to work just a bit harder to understand what's being said.

It's not just sound — "seeing" what you hear

Intuitively, you may think that the brain uses just the signal from the ear to figure out the meaning of the sound, but there's more to it! As the brain works to decode the sound signal (particularly sounds related to speech and language), the brain also relies on visual cues to understand what's being said. These visual cues can involve the speaker's facial expressions but more importantly how the speaker's lips move.

"But hold on," you may say. "I've never been trained to read lips!"

Well, yes and no. While you may never have received formal training in lip reading, you (and everyone else) have been doing it since the day you were born. These brain processes, whereby certain lip movements are matched up with certain sounds, are critical when children learn to understand and speak, and these links between certain sounds and lip movements are used by your brain all the time.

Still don't believe us? Imagine the situation of watching a movie where the audio track is a bit delayed relative to the visual images, so the lip movements and voice don't match up. It's completely distracting and annoying, right?

Or try to recall a situation where you've seen a foreign movie dubbed into your native language, but the dubbing hasn't been the best quality and the lip movements are completely off sync with the dubbed voice. Again, it's completely annoying, right?

This asynchrony is jarring because our brains routinely merge visual lip movements and speech sounds to decode the meaning of what was said.

A nice example of the brain's dependence on visual cues for decoding auditory signals has come up a lot during the COVID-19 pandemic, when everyone started wearing masks. During this period, we've been seeing patients who have suddenly noticed problems with understanding others and have been concerned that they have a problem with their hearing. The real cause in some cases is they've lost the visual cues that they've always depended on when hearing and understanding others.

Context matters

As the brain processes and decodes auditory signals, visual cues are key, but context matters as well. For example, if you hear the phrase, "It's raining, grab the . . .", your brain is already expecting the following word to be something like "umbrella."

Likewise, in a restaurant, if you hear the server say something to the effect of, "Would you like to hear the . . . of the day?" your brain will likely fill in the blank with a word like "specials." The point of these examples is to demonstrate that your brain is often already narrowing down what the auditory signal may be, based on the circumstances and the context of what's being said.

Pinpointing Where the System Can Break Down

When someone notices difficulties hearing and understanding speech, the problem can be with any of the essential pieces of hearing: sound, the ear, or the brain. In many cases, more than one piece is affected before communication problems become apparent. The following sections identify where breakdowns can occur.

When sound quality is poor

Quality matters. It may seem pretty obvious, but in the context of hearing, the quality of the incoming sound makes a huge difference. The poorer the sound quality is, the more the individual has to rely on the other essential pieces of the hearing system to work correctly for the word to be understandable. Lots of factors can affect the quality of spoken speech, including the following:

>> **Background noise:** Sounds such as other people talking in the same room, radio or TV sounds, and loud air conditioners can interfere and degrade the quality of the speech that you want to listen to.

>> **Room characteristics and acoustics:** Rooms with lots of hard surfaces tend to reflect sound, leading to constant reverberation and echoing that can degrade the quality of the incoming sound.

>> **Unfamiliar speakers:** Our brains are often attuned to hearing speech that we're most familiar with. Speech from someone you don't know or who has an unfamiliar accent will be of poorer quality, from your brain's perspective, than the voice of a close family member.

When the sound can't get in

The external and middle ear collect sound waves and convert these sound waves into a mechanical movement of the ear bones. Any physical processes that affect the transmission of these sound waves or the movement of the ear bones in the middle ear affect hearing and lead to what is called a *conductive hearing loss* — meaning that the sound can't be conducted into the inner ear (more on this in Chapter 7).

For the external ear, these obstacles can be attributed to

>> Ear wax (*cerumen*) that completely blocks the entire ear canal (more on this in Chapter 3)

>> External ear infections that lead to swelling of the external ear canal

>> Foreign objects in the ear canal, such as cotton from a cotton swab or a hearing aid ear dome stuck in the ear canal

For the middle ear, obstacles can include:

>> Holes in the eardrum from previous infection or trauma to the ear

>> Fluid in the middle ear from an ear infection, or nasal allergies or an upper respiratory tract infection (for example, a cold) that lead to swelling around the Eustachian tube opening (more on this in Chapter 3)

>> Diseases of the ear bones that lead to them stiffening in place (more on this in Chapter 3)

Problems of the external or middle ear that cause problems with hearing typically come on suddenly or are associated with pain, infections, or other symptoms.

When the inner ear garbles the encoding of sound

The inner ear is responsible for faithfully converting the mechanical movement of the ear bones that is transmitted to the cochlea into a precise electrical signal that goes to the brain. Those highly specialized hair cells in the cochlea, with their cilia, pull off this amazing feat. These sensory hair cells and other components of the inner ear can become damaged over time from various processes (see Chapter 3) and, unlike other cells of the body, can't regenerate. When this happens, the inner ear can still transmit a signal to the brain, but it is no longer a crystal clear and faithful encoding of the incoming sound.

REMEMBER

This is far and away the most common type of hearing loss that people experience, and this type of hearing loss is called a *sensorineural hearing loss,* meaning that the *sensory* hair cells and *neural* encoding of sound are impaired. Individuals with sensorineural hearing loss will note that speech often sounds unclear or as if the speaker is mumbling or garbling their words.

Nearly every person experiences sensorineural hearing loss over time; it comes on gradually and slowly over a period of decades. People in their 50s often begin noticing these hearing changes. Words may not sound as clear, and we need to occasionally ask people to repeat themselves. Chapter 3 covers this in more detail.

When the brain struggles to process sound

The ear encodes sound, but unless the brain effectively decodes the resulting signal, you aren't able to understand what's going on. Many people don't think about the brain decoding process, assuming that hearing is just about the ear. In reality, any process that adversely affects the brain can also adversely affect the decoding of sound and, hence, your ability to hear and understand the sounds around you.

Examples of what can affect the brain and, therefore, the brain's ability to process and decode sound include the following:

>> Concussions and post-concussive syndromes

>> Traumatic brain injury

>> Cognitive impairment and dementia

>> Other conditions or factors that affect thinking, concentration, and memory abilities such as attention deficit hyperactivity disorder, a stroke, drugs that may affect the brain, and even fatigue

REMEMBER

In general, anything that affects the brain's ability to think and concentrate also affects the brain's ability to process and decode auditory signals. This is because the decoding process of an auditory signal draws on the same areas of the brain that are needed for thinking and memory tasks. Some isolated conditions of the brain may affect only sound processing and are called *central auditory processing disorders*, but more often than not, such conditions are often also associated with other conditions affecting the brain.

Experiencing Trouble Hearing

People often begin to notice problems with hearing when one or, more commonly, two or more of the pieces of the hearing system break down (as noted earlier in the chapter, this could be the quality of the incoming sound, external/middle ear, inner ear, or the brain). There is some redundancy in our hearing system that often allows pieces of the system to help compensate for another part of the system, and hearing problems may not become markedly noticeable until two or more of these pieces of the system are having issues.

For example, a 75-year-old woman with some age-related sensorineural hearing loss may do fine when communicating with others when the sound quality is good (say her children speak with her face-to-face in a quiet room). In this case, even if a high-quality sound is slightly degraded during the inner ear's encoding process, the brain can still easily compensate during decoding.

In contrast, if the incoming sound quality is poor (say, when she's trying to hear others in a busy coffee shop) or if the visual cues of the speaker are taken away (such as when wearing a face mask), this woman may struggle with hearing others.

Likewise, someone with mild sensorineural hearing loss and early dementia may also struggle even under ideal listening conditions when the sound quality is good because of the combined effects of both the sensorineural hearing loss and the reduced ability of the brain to process sound related to dementia.

REMEMBER

Because we use both our ears and our brains to hear and there are redundancies built into the process, hearing loss is not always immediately evident to us. In fact, most people don't realize they have hearing loss or underestimate the extent of their hearing loss. Chapter 5 will explain why in more detail and review signs of hearing loss.

Each piece of the hearing system plays an important role in the ability to turn sound into meaning. By knowing how each piece functions and how all the pieces work together, you can better understand why you may be struggling with your hearing and what you can do about it.

As we discuss in Part 3, many of the strategies to help enhance your ability to hear and communicate effectively focus on trying to optimize these different pieces of the hearing system.

Chapter **3**

Looking at Types of Hearing Loss and Minimizing Risk

P roblems with hearing, as you find out in Chapter 2, can be caused by a whole range of different reasons ranging from poor sound quality to processes affecting the outer or middle ear, or conditions that affect the brain. But far and away, the most common cause of hearing problems among all of humanity is what has generally been called *age-related sensorineural hearing loss* (also referred to as age-related hearing loss or *presbycusis* in medical jargon).

This is the hearing loss that your grandfather has, your mother has, your uncle has, your friends have . . . and well, you get the point. How can this be so, you ask? How is it that everyone loses some hearing over time? Is there anything you can do to prevent this? This chapter gets into how this type of hearing loss happens and what can be done about it.

We also review other common conditions that can affect hearing. And you find out why hearing loss matters, not only to you, but to everyone else around you and society at large.

Discovering Why Hearing Gets Worse Over Time

At the most basic and fundamental level, hearing gets worse over time because many of the critical cells in the inner ear can't regenerate. That means once these cells become damaged, they can't always repair themselves, and if they die off, new ones don't pop up in their place.

Other parts of the body don't have this problem. For example, cells in your liver can regenerate, and the same goes for your muscle cells and even some types of brain cells. Scientists don't know yet why the cells in the inner ear appear to be the exception.

The important thing to note is that as these cells of the inner ear get progressively damaged over time, the result is the sensorineural hearing loss that is often seen with aging. The inner ear is responsible for faithfully converting sounds into a precise signal that goes to the brain, and this process depends on specialized cells in the cochlea.

Many of these highly specialized cells, particularly the sensory hair cells, can't regenerate after becoming damaged. When this happens, the inner ear can still transmit a signal to the brain, but it's no longer a crystal clear and faithful encoding of the incoming sound. People with this type of hearing loss, therefore, will notice that people's voices sound unclear or as if the speaker is mumbling.

Knowing the Causes of Hearing Loss Over Time

If some of the cells of the inner ear can't regenerate after being damaged, what in fact damages the cells in the first place? Unfortunately, a lot of different things can contribute to this, and for most people who develop hearing loss over time, it's not just one thing but a host of different things that leads to sensorineural hearing loss over time.

Biological aging processes

Why humans age at all is a daunting scientific question, and why cells in the inner ear age is no different. Many different processes that could affect the inner ear have been studied and proposed, and some of these include the following:

>> **Instability and progressive damage to the cell's DNA:** The DNA of a cell encodes the instructions to make the proteins that a cell needs to function.

>> **Dysfunction of mitochondria in the cells:** The *mitochondria* are the "power plants" of the cell that generate the energy needed by the cell to maintain function.

>> **Inflammation and other cellular processes:** Some processes can adversely affect how cells communicate with one another or the cell's ability to make the proteins necessary to function properly.

These are just a minuscule sample of some of the things that can lead to aging of the cells in the inner ear and that accumulate over time and damage the inner ear.

Cardiovascular risk factors

The cells in any part of the body need a blood supply to get oxygen and other substances (such as sugar and nutrients) essential to stay alive. The inner ear is no different, and this blood supply comes from a small network of blood vessels.

Lots of different things can adversely affect these microscopic blood vessels, and you probably won't be surprised to find out that these are the same things that are bad for the blood vessels that go to your brain and other parts of the body. Some of these risk factors include:

>> Smoking

>> High blood pressure

>> High cholesterol

>> Diabetes

Many of these risk factors may sound familiar because you've likely heard them before from your doctors and other sources. Namely, these are the same cardiovascular risk factors we all want to address to avoid developing conditions like heart disease and strokes. These same risk factors that can damage the blood vessels feeding the brain and other parts of the body can also damage the fine blood vessels that go to the inner ear. Injured blood vessels here mean less blood supply to the inner ear and ultimately to damaged and dysfunctional cells of the inner ear.

Genetics

It may not be much of a surprise to you that your genetics can affect the damage that occurs to your inner ear over time. Your genetics, or your DNA, determines a lot about how your cells and body function, particularly in response to other things like noise, biological aging processes, and smoking, which can affect the ear as well. Read on to see how some of these genetic factors can influence your risk of developing hearing loss over time.

Biological sex

Your genetics, of course, determine whether you're biologically a female (sex chromosomes XX) or male (sex chromosomes XY). This biological determination then affects a whole slew of different hormones and other processes in the body. Estrogen is the key sex hormone that is made much more in women than men. Scientists now think that estrogen may also affect the inner ear and help protect it from damage over time. This observation would go a long way toward explaining why hearing loss is much more commonly seen in men than women.

Skin color

The color of your skin is in large part determined by how much melanin your skin makes, which is dictated by your DNA. *Melanin* is the pigment in your skin cells that gives the skin its color. Lots of melanin means darker skin, and less melanin means paler skin. Interestingly, there's also some melanin pigment in your inner ear, and the amount corresponds to how much melanin your skin makes.

Amazingly, it appears that this melanin in the inner ear also helps protect the inner ear from various sources of damage. It appears to be similar to melanin's role in the skin, whereby melanin helps the skin cells combat the harmful effects of the sun's radiation on the skin. People with darker skin are less likely to develop melanoma skin cancers than those with paler skin.

These scientific findings help explain epidemiological data that have accumulated over the years about hearing loss. In these studies, skin color consistently appears to be very strongly related to risk of hearing loss. In general, individuals with lighter skin had much higher rates of hearing loss, and other studies suggest that lighter-skinned people are much more susceptible to noise exposure damaging their hearing.

Other genetic factors

Sex and skin color are some of the key genetic-related factors, but there are a lot more. Genetic characteristics involving genes related to inflammation, detoxification systems of the cells, and how cells join together all appear to have a role in hearing loss. Some of these genes seem to affect how well the cells in your ear can deal with the biological aging processes described earlier in this chapter, while others may affect how your inner ear responds to insults like noise and some medications (see the section "Medications" later in the chapter) linked to hearing loss.

REMEMBER

The key thing to remember is that no single gene determines whether you'll get hearing loss. Hundreds of different genes seemingly all interact with each other and other factors (such as noise) that affect your risk of hearing loss over time.

Note that from a genetic perspective, hearing loss that develops over time is very different than sensorineural hearing losses that occur in young children or in families with a strong family history of hearing loss that occurs in early adulthood. In these relatively rare cases, occasionally a single gene can be responsible for the hearing loss.

Minimizing Your Risk for Hearing Loss

You may be familiar with the Serenity Prayer, which goes like this: "God, grant me the serenity to accept the things I cannot change, the courage to change the things I can, and the wisdom to know the difference." Well, you can actually apply the Serenity Prayer to hearing loss.

Many of the most common causes of hearing loss, as we describe earlier in this chapter, fall into the "cannot change" category. Epidemiological studies in the past have shown that age, sex, and race are the dominant and most important risk factors that determine a person's chances of developing hearing loss over time. In this sense, your chronological age is a general marker of the biological processes of aging, sex is linked with estrogen and its protective role in the inner ear, and race is a rough marker of someone skin's color and, hence, melanin in the inner ear. Needless to say, these are things that we can't directly change or influence.

In contrast, you do have some control of these other factors.

Noise exposure

This is far and away the most important factor that you can control to minimize your risk of hearing loss over time. Recall that the impact of noise on the ears is cumulative, meaning it's generally not one event (short of something as loud as hearing a gunshot right next to your ear) that dictates how noise impacts your ear. Instead, it's all the little decisions and habits that accumulate over a lifetime that dictate how noise affects your hearing.

To put it bluntly, loud noises are not good for the inner ear. Here's why:

Loud noises = Really intense air vibrations shaking the eardrum and middle ear bones = Really strong fluid waves being transmitted to the inner ear from the middle ear = Sensory hair cells in the ear being shaken really, really hard

Things that get shaken really hard can get damaged and broken. The same is true of the structures in the inner ear.

REMEMBER

What can you do about it? At the personal level, the best general rule of thumb to remember on a daily basis is this:

If you have to raise your voice to be heard by someone at arm's length, the environment is noisy enough to hurt your ears.

In these cases, move away from the noise if you can, or if you can't, make sure to use some sort of ear protection (earplugs that go in your ear or noise-canceling headphones or earmuffs).

For example, imagine that you're in the backyard and the grass is up to your knees. You need to mow. But a lawnmower makes a racket, and you'd reach that noise threshold: You'd need to raise your voice to be heard. In this case, you could use earplugs or earmuffs to lessen the noise. Alternatively, if someone else is mowing your backyard (preferably with ear protection), move far enough away from the lawnmower so the noise won't be loud enough where you would have trouble holding a conversation with someone at arm's length.

TIP

There's a lot more to noise prevention, or what are collectively called hearing conservation programs, particularly related to federal workplace regulations, but these are beyond the scope of this book. A great resource for further reading is: www.cdc.gov/niosh/topics/noise/default.html and www.dangerous decibels.org.

The key thing to note is that noise damage to the ear can accumulate over time and work in tandem with other factors that can hurt your ears. Hence, the effects of attending a series of rock concerts in your 20s may not be readily apparent until decades later.

Knowing when to use ear protection

You may be wondering at this point when you need to use ear protection and when you don't throughout your day. For example, you may be periodically in situations throughout the day where you have to raise your voice to be heard with someone at arm's length. Do you have to use ear protection all the time in these settings?

DO I STILL NEED TO WORRY ABOUT NOISE PROTECTION IF I ALREADY HAVE SOME HEARING LOSS?

There is a common misconception that once you have hearing loss, you don't need to worry about noise as much and don't need protection. The truth is exactly the opposite! You need hearing protection now more than ever to preserve what hearing you still have.

Sound occurs on a spectrum of soft to loud volume. Hearing loss is a phenomenon that changes our ability to discriminate sounds on the softer end of that spectrum but what is loud and dangerous to our ears does NOT change at all. Even with hearing loss, dangerously loud sounds can and will damage your hearing without protection.

If you already have a hearing loss and are concerned about using protective earmuffs since you won't be able to hear as well, you can look for amplified hearing protective earmuffs that amplify some sound to help you hear while providing protection from dangerously loud sounds. If you wear hearing aids, they can be worn under regular hearing protective earmuffs, but you may need to consult a professional to help you optimize the settings.

The answer is an unsatisfying: "It depends." The reason for this equivocal answer is that whether noise damages your ears or not is related to both the intensity (loudness) of the noise and the duration to which you're exposed to it. A gunshot next to your ear for a split second is loud enough to damage your ears permanently. In contrast, being exposed to the noise on a busy subway platform would take hundreds of hours of exposure to damage your ears.

The federal government has specific recommendations for suggested maximum daily exposure to occupational noise based on how loud the noise is, but these guidelines aren't really practical outside the workplace setting. The best general guidance remains the rule of thumb above. Namely, if you have to raise your voice to be heard at arm's length, the environment is loud enough to hurt your ears. In these situations, you'll want to minimize your time in such environments or use ear protection.

Avoiding noise exposure from headphone use

You may also be wondering about using headphones and earphones and whether these could be too loud for your ears as well. In short, the answer is unequivocally "Yes" when they are turned up too loud and for too long. Here are a few practical tips to avoid this situation:

>> Use over-the-ear headphones whenever possible rather than in-the-ear earbuds. Over the ear headphones block out more of the ambient noise so you won't have to turn the volume as high.

>> Use headphone or earbuds with a noise cancellation feature. This feature also allows you to avoid having to turn the volume as loud.

>> For headphones or earbuds with a smartphone, use the smartphone's built-in programs to restrict the sound output to safe levels (less than 85 dB). Both Android and Apple phones now have such programs in their Settings menu that will guide you through how to choose the level.

>> Use headphones that have a built-in volume limiter. These headphones are often designed for kids so that there's no way the sound can be turned too loud.

>> Use your earbuds or headphones for no more than 60 minutes at a time and give your ears a break between periods of use.

Keeping your ear heart-healthy

You may have heard the phrase, What's good for the heart is good for the brain. Well, that also extends to the ear: What's good for the heart is good for your hearing. You may already be trying your best to follow many of these tips because you want to avoid a heart attack or stroke, not realizing you're also helping to reduce your risk for hearing loss!

These factors include the same things that you may already know are important for preventing cardiovascular disease. Cardiovascular diseases include a group of related diseases that affect the blood vessels supplying your heart, brain, and other parts of your body — including your inner ear.

TIP

Some of these tips are summarized in the following list, and a great resource for further reading is at the CDC's website at www.cdc.gov/heartdisease/prevention.htm.

>> Choose healthy foods and drinks. This includes limiting sodium (salt) and alcohol and avoiding foods high in saturated fats.

>> Get regular physical activity and exercise every day.

>> Refrain from cigarette smoking.

>> Take charge of any medical conditions that you may have that can lead to cardiovascular disease, such as high cholesterol, high blood pressure, and diabetes.

Considering Other Conditions That Affect Hearing

While aging, noise, and cardiovascular problems can contribute to sensorineural hearing loss in adults, a variety of other medical diseases and conditions either cause or are often related to hearing loss. Some of these you undoubtedly have heard of, while others are less common but are important to mention because they may require further medical evaluation.

The almighty ear infection

Alright, everyone at some point in time has heard of someone getting an ear infection, but what does this mean, what causes it, and what can you do about it? An ear infection can actually involve any of the three parts of the ear (external, middle, and inner; see Chapter 2).

Infections of the external or middle ear can generally just lead to a temporary conductive hearing loss until the infection resolves whereas infections of the inner ear often lead to a permanent sensorineural hearing loss.

External ear infections

An external ear infection involves the skin of the ear canal becoming infected and is often known as "swimmer's ear" because it can be triggered by too much moisture in the ear canal. When this happens, it's easier for bacteria to grow in the ear canal.

Another common cause is when someone sticks their finger or a cotton swab in the ear and inadvertently traumatizes the skin, leading to an infection.

External ear infections often come with pain, swelling, and drainage from the ear and may occasionally be accompanied by a temporary decrease in hearing related to swelling or infected material in the ear canal preventing sound from getting to the eardrum (known as conductive hearing loss). Once this infection resolves, the transient conductive hearing loss resolves as well.

If you think you have an external ear infection, you'll want to see your primary care doctor or an ENT (ear, nose, and throat specialist; see Chapter 6) because you may need the ear cleaned and antibiotic ear drops or pills.

Middle ear infections

Middle ear infections generally occur when fluid accumulates in the middle ear space and gets infected leading to a temporary conductive hearing loss.

Huh?

Didn't we say before that the middle ear space is filled with air? How can fluid possibly get there?

THE ROLE OF THE MYSTERIOUS EUSTACHIAN TUBE

TECHNICAL
STUFF

To understand how this can happen, we have to briefly pause here and introduce one more part of the ear that's critical to know about before we can discuss middle ear infections. The *Eustachian tube* is a fancy term for a narrow tube that connects the middle ear space to the very back of the nose (see Chapter 2). This tube is critically important because it's the structure that allows air to move back and forth between the middle ear and the outside environment.

Why is this relevant and what does it have to do with ear infections, you ask?

Well, the air in the middle ear space is constantly getting absorbed by the lining of the middle ear, which is similar to the lining of the lungs. The cells of this lining are designed to absorb air. The Eustachian tube, therefore, allows "new" air to get in from the outside to replenish the air in the middle ear as it is gradually absorbed over the course of the day.

THE HIDDEN CULPRIT OF MIDDLE EAR INFECTIONS

TECHNICAL
STUFF

Okay, okay, you're still probably asking what this possibly has to do with a middle ear infection.

Imagine what would happen if the Eustachian tube weren't open and air couldn't get to the ear to replenish the air that's getting absorbed. In this case, the middle ear space would rapidly become a vacuum (in other words, there wouldn't be enough air pressure) as the air would be absorbed by the lining of the middle ear. As you may have heard before, "Nature abhors a vacuum," and it's true here as well! With a vacuum in the middle ear, the middle ear space gets filled with fluid that's sucked out of the cells lining the middle ear. It sounds a bit crazy, but it's true.

Fluid collecting in the middle ear can lead to a sense of pressure and fullness in the ear as well as a temporary hearing loss as sounds can't be transmitted effectively to the inner ear through the fluid. If the fluid gets infected, you'll also notice lots of pain, which may be accompanied by a fever. If you think you have a middle ear infection, you'll definitely want to see a doctor because you may need oral antibiotics to treat the ear infection.

Middle ear infections can most often be triggered by getting a cold or having nasal allergies. In these cases, the lining of the nose and the back of the throat can get swollen and inflamed, which blocks the opening around the Eustachian tube, preventing air from getting back and forth.

The good news is that the conductive hearing loss caused by a middle ear infection is only temporary until the infection resolves and the fluid in the middle ear drains out through the Eustachian tube.

Inner ear infections

Unlike external and middle ear infections, which are relatively common and have symptoms that resolve after being treated, inner ear infections are relatively rare and far more dangerous to your hearing. The inner ear is generally resistant to ear infections since it's hard for bacteria and viruses to get into and infect the fluid of the inner ear. Unfortunately, while it's rare, scientists think about 1 in 10,000 to 50,000 people a year get inner ear infections.

In these cases, doctors think that most commonly some type of virus manages to get into the inner ear and damage the inner ear, leading to a sudden loss of hearing. Not surprisingly, it's called a *sudden sensorineural hearing loss* (SSNHL — ear doctors have absolutely no imagination or creativity when it comes to naming diseases!).

WARNING

SSNHL is an urgent medical condition. The earlier it's diagnosed and treated (ideally within three to five days), the better the chance of some recovery of hearing. The key thing to note about an SSNHL is that the hearing loss comes on suddenly — over a period of minutes — and often completely out of the blue in just one ear. (In contrast, hearing loss from an external or middle ear infection is not nearly so sudden or severe, is often accompanied by other symptoms, and may affect both ears.)

Earwax — ick!

Ahhh . . . we've all heard of earwax before and the jokes that come along with it. But does earwax actually affect your hearing, and do you need to do anything about it?

Earwax explained

First, just to get the facts straight, earwax (or cerumen) is a naturally occurring oily substance that the skin of the outer portion of the ear canal produces. This oil helps protect the thin skin of the ear canal. Some people have a more oily, sticky type of earwax, while for others it can be dried and harder. Both are normal.

The most important thing to know is that the ear actually has a self-cleaning mechanism where the ear naturally expels and gets rid of the earwax by itself. This happens because as new skin cells are formed in the ear canal, they naturally help push the old skin cells mixed up with earwax out of the ear.

Opening and closing the jaw also naturally leads to a pumping-like motion of the outer portion of the ear canal that is held open by cartilage that sits just behind the jaw joint. These movements help expel this old skin and earwax out of the ear. Every time you shower and dry around your ear with a towel, little bits of earwax are likely coming out on their own, unbeknownst to you! Yuck!

Why earwax gets backed up

That being said, occasionally earwax can get backed up and start accumulating in the ear canal, leading to an obstruction of the ear canal. This most commonly occurs in certain instances:

REMEMBER

» **If you use a cotton swab to clean your ears:** Cotton swabs, despite their appearance, aren't meant to go in the ear canal. When they do, you risk plunging some of the earwax back into your ear and impeding the natural outbound migration of the earwax.

» **If you have very small or narrow ear canals:** Some individuals naturally have smaller ear canals that make it harder for earwax to get out on its own. As you get older, the outer portion of the ear canal that's held open by cartilage also gets weaker. This can lead to the outer portion of the ear canal partially collapsing, thereby allowing earwax to more easily accumulate.

» **If you have skin conditions around the ear that lead to increased skin flaking or excess earwax production:** Certain skin conditions such as eczema (an itchy inflammation of the skin) can also affect the ears.

Interestingly, earwax in and of itself rarely affects your hearing too much. To do so, the *entire* ear canal has to be blocked by a plug of earwax to prevent all sound from getting to your eardrum. If you think you have earwax blocking your hearing, you should see your primary care doctor or an ENT (see Chapter 6). The key thing to note is that any hearing loss caused by ear wax is purely temporary until the ear wax is removed.

Diseases of the ear

A lot of diseases that can affect the ear and hearing are rare. We go over just a few of the relatively more frequent ones here that you may occasionally hear of (ha-ha!). If any of these symptoms seem familiar to you, you'll want to see your doctor.

>> **Meniere's disease:** This is a condition that typically affects just one ear and can lead to sudden episodes of decreased hearing and buzzing in one ear, a sense of pressure in the affected ear, and often a sense of spinning (also called vertigo) that can last for up to an hour. These episodes often come out of the blue, and after they resolve, individuals often feel fine again. Scientists think the condition may be caused by too much fluid building up in the cochlea. Treatments include staying on a low-salt diet and taking a *diuretic* (a medicine that regulates how your body handles water) and other medicines. Over time, Meniere's disease can sometimes lead to a permanent sensorineural hearing loss.

>> **Otosclerosis:** *Otosclerosis* is a condition that occasionally runs in families (there's somewhat of a genetic component) where the ear bone in the middle ear that pushes into the inner ear (the stapes bone) can become fused and stiffened in place. When this happens, sound can't be transmitted effectively through the middle ear leading to a conductive hearing loss (see Chapter 2). Individuals notice a progressive hearing loss in the affected ear, and over time otosclerosis can affect one or both ears. This condition is generally easily diagnosed by an ENT based on hearing and other diagnostic tests. Treatments include hearing aids or different surgical approaches to releasing the ear bone or placing a surgically implantable hearing device that can transmit sound directly to the cochlear and bypass the "stuck" ear bones (see Chapter 12).

Medications

Most medications don't hurt hearing. However, a couple of classes of medications are recognized to be particularly *ototoxic* (that is, potentially damaging to the inner ear) and are important to be mindful of. These include

>> **Aminoglycoside antibiotics:** These are a class of antibiotics often ending with the suffix -micin or -mycin (neomycin, gentamicin, and so on) that can be toxic to the inner ear. Doctors generally avoid prescribing them since it's well recognized that these drugs can hurt the inner ear. Occasionally, these drugs may be prescribed when someone has a severe infection for which other safer antibiotics won't work. If so, these medications are often only administered in the hospital setting because they have to be given intravenously.

You'll also occasionally see these antibiotics used in ointments or drops, but these formulations aren't likely to affect your ear because the medication can't get to your inner ear. For instance, an antibiotic first-aid ointment with neomycin used on a cut on your knee won't get to your inner ear.

>> **Platinum-based chemotherapy cancer drugs:** This class of drugs often used to treat cancers (most commonly, cisplatin and carboplatin) can also have the side effect of damaging the inner ear and your hearing. Patients who need these drugs to treat cancer may have their hearing routinely monitored to check for adverse effects.

Causing Tinnitus

Buzzzzzzz . . .

Eeeeeeeee . . .

Ever hear either of those sounds transiently in your ear as you've been lost in your thoughts in a quiet room? Most commonly, the sound is described as being a high-pitched whistling or a chirping sound. If so, you've experienced tinnitus!

Tinnitus is really, really common, and it's the perception of hearing a sound in your head that's not generated by an external source (in other words, the buzzing's not coming from your refrigerator or other appliance). Almost everyone experiences tinnitus at some point in their life, often for just a few seconds or minutes, and it's completely normal every now and then.

But when tinnitus lasts for longer (weeks to months), there may be other things causing this sound to occur. Hearing loss is the most common cause of tinnitus, but other conditions can contribute as well. The important thing to note is that tinnitus does NOT cause hearing loss but instead is a common symptom associated with hearing loss.

Tinnitus explained

Why does this happen, you ask? Well, the sound you're hearing with tinnitus is actually generated not by the ears but actually by the hearing part of the brain, which is called the *auditory cortex.* This part of your brain sits on either side of your head just above your ears and works to process the sounds you hear.

The reason that this part of the brain may occasionally make this sound has a lot to do with how the auditory cortex is connected to other parts of the brain and body. For example, the auditory cortex has neural (nerve) connections with

>> **The inner ear (cochlea):** The inner ear is constantly sending sound signals to the auditory cortex, where the signals are processed and decoded (see Chapter 2).

>> **Sensory nerves and muscles in your head and neck:** Connections between these areas and the auditory cortex may have to do with the fact that the sounds we hear often affect how we move and control these areas of the body.

>> **Areas of the brain that affect your emotions:** Nerve connections here between the auditory cortex and emotional areas of the brain likely explain how sounds can often affect our emotions (imagine hearing a sad song).

Often when people notice tinnitus, it's because one of these other areas of the brain or body has changed the level of input or feedback that is being given to the auditory cortex. When this happens, the auditory cortex in turn may change its level of brain activity, which leads to the perception of tinnitus. Most often, the brain then readjusts the activity and the tinnitus subsides after a period of time. This period of time can be minutes to months depending on the severity of the underlying triggers that led to the tinnitus.

Tinnitus triggers

Potential things that can trigger tinnitus. Check out the following table:

Source	Potential Triggers
Ear	Any process that affects the sound being sent from the ear to the auditory cortex. This can be sensorineural hearing loss, conductive hearing loss (for example, a cold leading to fluid in the middle ear), and exposure to a loud noise (for example, listening to music too loudly can stun the inner ear and affect the signal sent to the brain).
Sensory nerves and muscles of the head and neck	Arthritis or cervical disk problems of the neck, muscle stiffness in the neck, temporomandibular joint (jaw joint) problems.
Emotional and other areas of the brain	Feeling stressed, anxious, or tired; migraine headaches; concussions; or traumatic brain injury.

Most often, tinnitus just happens sporadically and is generally considered normal because it's related to how the brain and ear are all wired together. If you have tinnitus that's constantly getting worse, accompanied by worsening hearing or balance problems, or causing you a lot of stress and anxiety, you'll want to consult with your primary care doctor or an ENT.

Chapter **4**

Realizing What You Lose When You Can't Hear

You might wonder: If almost everyone is going to experience some degree of hearing loss over time, how could it be that important?

This "safety in numbers" mentality may make sense at first but quickly falls apart with a bit more careful thought. At its foundation, your ability to effortlessly hear and understand others is what connects you to everyone around you. Loss of this sense forces the brain to constantly struggle with interpreting sounds, and what was once effortless is now a constant challenge.

Over the past decade scientists have begun to understand how hearing loss that develops over time can affect the body and the brain. In this chapter, you find out more about why your hearing matters and why scientists now think hearing loss may be the most important, potentially treatable risk factor for dementia in later life.

Communicating Is Like a Game of Catch

We like to compare hearing to the iconic American pastime of two people playing catch. One person throws the ball, the other catches it and then throws the ball back, and the cycle repeats itself over and over.

Having a conversation with someone is similar. One person says something, the other person listens (and "catches" the spoken words), says something back, and the cycle continues, sometimes for hours! This process is often effortless, and in many cases, we take for granted how we can understand what was said and reply instantaneously.

Hearing loss affects how well you can play catch

What does this have to do with hearing? Well, imagine a game of catch where someone is constantly dropping the ball when trying to catch it. The natural back and forth rhythm of catching and throwing is missing, there are a lot of pauses, and the game takes a bit more work and isn't as much fun.

Having a hearing loss affects your ability to catch words in a conversation in a similar way and can make back-and-forth conversations more effortful and perhaps not as enjoyable. With a hearing loss, the inner ear is no longer able to send sounds clearly to the brain, making it harder for your brain to understand and "catch" what was spoken.

In this case, you may still be able to hear what is being said, but the brain has to work harder (and may take a bit longer) to decode the sound signal and understand what was said. Your brain may have to use other clues to decode the garbled sound signal, such as relying on visual lip cues from the speaker and using context about the conversation. This process takes time and mental energy and can affect how well you're able to understand what was spoken and engage in a conversation.

Why playing catch is sometimes easier or harder

Okay, we promise that this is the last time we use the "catch" analogy, but we can't help ourselves since we're both baseball fans and the analogy (we think! . . . hope?) works here.

Imagine a situation where someone who is not a great ball player receives an easy lob from a friend. The ball is aimed perfectly, tossed at just the right speed, and just plain easy to catch. Even though the person isn't very good at catching, the ball can still be caught.

This situation is equivalent to communicating in a quiet room with a familiar speaker. With no background noise and just a single, familiar speaker, the voice you want to hear comes in clearly to the ear. In these situations, even if you were to have some hearing loss and the signal being sent to the brain was slightly distorted by the impaired inner ear, your brain could still easily decode and "catch" the signal, particularly since your brain is attuned to that familiar person's voice.

In contrast, imagine instead that you're in a crowded, noise-filled restaurant and speaking with someone you've just met. In this case, the speaker's voice may already be muffled before it even reaches your ear. With hearing loss, your inner ear then further garbles this sound during the encoding process, and by the time your brain receives the signal, the sound has been thoroughly distorted and is much harder to decode and understand. This would be the equivalent of trying to catch a ball that is thrown very fast and off target. Someone really good at catch — and someone with good hearing — may not have a problem, but if you're not so good at catch — or you have hearing loss — you're going to struggle.

This analogy also applies to when there are multiple speakers at once (for example, at a cocktail party or a meeting table), which would be equivalent to trying catch a series of balls thrown by different people nearly at the same time. Again, if you're good at catch — or your hearing is good — you may not have much of a problem, but you may struggle with a hearing loss.

People with hearing loss may also notice that certain voice registers (a high-pitched woman's voice versus a low-pitched man's voice, for example) may be easier or harder to understand. This can happen based on your pattern or degree of hearing loss at different frequencies of sound. We talk about this more in Chapter 7.

Communication and hearing loss in critical situations

If we always communicated in a quiet room face-to-face with a familiar speaker, everything would be a lot easier for people with hearing loss. Unfortunately, while this may be the case at home, this certainly isn't the case in other environments when effective communication may affect our livelihood or our health.

Hearing loss at work

Effective spoken communication is often critical for occupations requiring interaction with others. Not being able to hear others in a virtual or in-person meeting, communicate with a coworker on the phone, or interact with a customer over lunch are all examples of situations where hearing loss can affect a person's ability to carry out their job effectively.

Economic research on this topic is sparse but is consistent with what you'd expect. Individuals with hearing loss appear to be at greater risk of being unemployed or underemployed (working less than they would like) compared to those with normal hearing. The research doesn't have the precision to look at more subtle outcomes such as the risk of being passed up for a promotion, but these outcomes may be even more strongly related to hearing loss and its effects on communication.

In Parts 3 and 4, you can find out more about the different strategies to address communication issues in the workplace and your legal rights under the Americans with Disabilities Act.

Hearing loss in healthcare interactions

It's hard to imagine a more important time when you would want to ensure you're understanding what is being said than when discussing your health with a healthcare provider. Explanations about a medical condition, instructions for how to take a medication, and discussions about what to expect with a medical procedure generally all take place via spoken communication. While we would hope that all clinicians are adept at good communication practices and know how to optimally communicate with patients who have hearing loss, we know this is often not the case.

Our research studying healthcare outcomes of adults with and without hearing loss has shown that those individuals with hearing loss consistently have worse healthcare outcomes, including higher medical care costs, greater risk of requiring hospitalization, and longer hospital stays. Some of these outcomes may be related to poor communication between patients and their healthcare providers, which can have subtle but significant effects on health.

For example, imagine a patient who didn't correctly hear their physician's instructions at a routine medical visit about changing their dose on a blood pressure medication. A few weeks later, the patient has an adverse medical event related to elevated blood pressure.

Alternatively, imagine a hospitalized patient who, because of hearing loss, can't easily communicate with their nurse or doctor and as a result, gets disoriented and delirious from lack of stimulation in the hospital setting.

These situations could both be directly related to hearing loss and impaired communication leading to adverse health effects. Parts 3 and 4 tell you more about how to optimize communication in these healthcare settings.

Watching for a Reduction in Social Interaction

We often take it for granted, but our daily social interactions with friends at the coffeeshop or a short chat with the postal carrier or the checkout clerk at the grocery store all depend on effective spoken communication. It's sort of like having to play multiple short games of catch with different people every day! (Sorry — we had to sneak in the catch analogy one last time!)

When these interactions become harder due to hearing loss, though, researchers have found that people may increasingly start limiting their social interactions to avoid the embarrassment, frustration, and fatigue that come with having difficulty understanding others. Outings become less frequent or less enjoyable, and certain places may be entirely avoided (such as loud restaurants and live theater).

This decrease in social interactions can often come on subtly and insidiously over time. For example, a person with hearing loss may start with turning down one social invitation to dinner, but then over time, this effect can cascade as that missed dinner leads to fewer interactions and, in turn, other missed invitations and opportunities to get together with others.

For individuals with a partner, the effects of hearing loss on the individual can also often extend to the partner. One individual's reluctance to go out can affect the other's social interactions as well, and researchers have found that this can lead to what has been called a "third-party disability." In this case, one person's hearing loss (disability) has carryover effects on a third party (the spouse, partner, or potentially other close family members or friends).

Importantly, as we discuss later in this chapter, researchers and physicians now know that maintaining rich social interactions with others is hugely important for our mental, emotional, cognitive, and physical health. Humans are social creatures by nature, and these constant social interactions help keep our brains mentally nimble and stimulated. Parts 3 and 4 discuss strategies you can use to keep these social interactions going strong!

Monitoring Mental and Emotional Health

Social interactions are important, but researchers also now understand that loneliness is a related but distinct concept that may be even more critical for mental and emotional health and may be one of the most important factors contributing to poor health outcomes as we grow older. First, we break down what loneliness is and how it matters, and then we connect it to hearing loss.

What is loneliness?

You might assume that being lonely relates to how social you are. But that's not necessarily so.

Social interactions or your social network are generally *objective* indicators of your level of social connectedness (or alternatively, social isolation). In fact, researchers count the number of people in someone's social circle and the number of outings with friends and relatives and find, not surprisingly, that on average, a greater number of social interactions is generally linked with people being happier and healthier.

But, wait, there's more to the story!

Unlike your number of social interactions, which you can consider to be an *objective* measure of your social connectedness, loneliness is a *subjective* indicator of how you *feel* about your social connections. Someone can have lots of social outings but still feel incredibly lonely because they have trouble communicating with others and feel left out of conversations.

On the flip side, someone with seemingly few social connections (perhaps just a spouse and a close family member or friend) may not feel lonely at all because of the depth of these relationships.

Another way of thinking about these concepts is that your number of social interactions reflects the *quantity* of your social connectedness while whether you feel lonely or not reflects the *quality* of those social connections.

How loneliness hurts your health

Researchers believe that loneliness may be one of the most important factors affecting our mental, cognitive, and physical health as we get older.

WARNING

To put it bluntly, loneliness is really bad for us, and individuals who are lonely are much more likely to develop a range of poor health outcomes including depression, dementia, and even earlier death. Scientists believe that loneliness can directly affect our health by increasing the level of inflammation in the body, which is a type of stress response that can damage our organs over time. Loneliness also may contribute to increased feelings of depression and anxiety over time, which takes a toll on our mental health.

In this sense, scientists estimate that chronic loneliness is more dangerous to our health than obesity and is roughly equivalent to smoking 15 cigarettes per day!

Looking at hearing loss and loneliness

At this point, you may be wondering why loneliness is relevant to hearing loss. Well, researchers are increasingly understanding that hearing loss may be an important factor that increases your chance of having chronic feelings of loneliness.

Namely, individuals with hearing loss may still indeed have social connections, but the quality of these social interactions may not be great if the individual is embarrassed or struggles with communicating in these social interactions. Being out to dinner with friends at a restaurant should be fun, but it may not be if you're constantly stressed about missing out on what was said and feeling left out.

At this point, if you're nodding your head and realizing that this may be what you're experiencing now and perhaps have been dealing with in silence for years, you're not alone! As clinicians, we talk with people routinely facing such struggles who are often hesitant to voice their concerns to others or don't know what to do. The good news is that you're reading this book now. In Parts 3 and 4 of this book, we review the strategies and technologies you can use to deal with hearing loss and to limit its impact on your ability to connect with others.

Losing Physical Abilities

Researchers now believe that hearing loss may also be linked to a decline of physical function — for example, maintaining your balance and being able to get around and take care of yourself. Studies have even shown that over time, older adults with hearing loss are more likely than those without hearing loss to eventually require a skilled nursing facility, potentially because they can't easily take care of their everyday needs.

How hearing affects your physical abilities

How are hearing loss and a decrease in physical abilities such as your walking speed connected? They may be related because of the effects that hearing loss has on social isolation, loneliness, and dementia, as we discuss earlier in this chapter. These things can all contribute subtly to poorer physical health over time as people are less likely to go out and become increasingly isolated at home. Over time, this can lead to our bodies becoming deconditioned and more physically frail.

How hearing affects your balance

Hearing loss can also increase your risk of losing your balance or having a fall. How's this, you say? Well, while our brains are ultimately responsible for allowing us to maintain our balance and walk around, the brain relies on several factors to do this well:

>> **Vision:** It seems obvious, of course, but your brain needs to see what's around you to allow you to move around.

>> **Blood output from your heart:** Moving takes oxygen and blood flow!

>> **Touch sensation and feeling in the feet and legs:** Your brain needs to be able to "feel" the surface you're walking on.

>> **Muscles and joints:** You need your legs and body to keep working well.

>> **Vestibular balance system:** How balance works (see the nearby sidebar, "Vestibular balance — The forgotten sixth sense," for more on this system).

>> **Hearing:** Okay, you knew we were going to say this.

Hmm . . . how does your brain need hearing to maintain balance? Well, imagine you're walking down a crowded city street with lots of other people. Now imagine doing this in total silence. It would be quite a different experience, and you may say it would even be nice, but in reality, all the sounds coming at you can help cue you in to what's around you and what to expect. Hearing the subtle sounds of people walking up behind you, your own footsteps hitting the sidewalk, and the rush of a car driving by all helps your brain anticipate and navigate the environment safely.

Researchers now believe these auditory (sound) cues may be really important for helping us maintain our balance effectively, particularly if one or more of the other systems the brain relies on isn't working as well. For example, your hearing may not be as critical for balance when you're young and healthy, but if you have poor vision, lack of feeling in your feet, or arthritic knees, hearing may play a critical role in maintaining your balance.

While research clearly shows that individuals with hearing loss compared to those with normal hearing are more likely to report having a fall or losing their balance, there's also evidence suggesting that strategies to give your ears more sound input (such as hearing aids and cochlear implants) may decrease this risk. You can find out more about these options later in this book.

VESTIBULAR BALANCE — THE FORGOTTEN SIXTH SENSE

People often naturally think that we have just five senses — hearing, vision, touch, taste, and smell. But what's often forgotten is the vestibular or balance system! What the heck is this? Well, it's the sense that allows your brain to know whether your body is turning, moving, falling, or jumping.

The inner ear contains the cochlea, which is the organ that converts sound waves into a signal that can go to the brain. The inner ear, though, also contains the vestibular system, which is comprised of a set of semicircular bony canals and the vestibule. The semicircular canals can detect when the head is turning, while the vestibule can detect vertical (such as falling) and linear (such as, accelerating in a car) motions.

Along with your other senses, the vestibular system allows your brain to understand where your body is in space and coordinate your body and eye movements. Medical conditions involving the vestibular system can lead to a sense of constant imbalance, vertigo (a sense of everything spinning around you even though you're still), and problems with maintaining your gaze when moving around (your vestibular system helps control your eye movements when your head is moving). Because the inner ear contains both the cochlea and vestibular balance systems, some diseases and medical conditions (for example, Meniere's disease) can adversely affect both the hearing and balance systems.

Dealing with a Decline in Cognitive Function

At some point, you may have come across information suggesting that hearing loss is a risk factor for dementia. Or perhaps you've unfortunately come across a predatory hearing aid advertisement claiming that you have to get hearing aids to prevent dementia. If you're wondering whether there's any actual scientific evidence underlying this information and what it means to you, you've come to the right place!

What are cognition and dementia?

First, we start with the basics. *Cognition* refers to your thinking and memory abilities. There are different aspects to cognition, and these include such areas as processing speed (for example, how quickly you can sort a deck of cards into the different suits), memory, math-related skills, and verbal language ability (for instance, being able to understand a complex written passage).

As we age, it's normal for our ability in some of these cognitive areas (such as processing speed and memory) to decline while others stay the same or even improve (such as math skills or verbal language ability). We may never seem to remember where we placed our keys but have absolutely no problem reading a dense history book or medical journal.

Dementia, on the other hand, is definitely not normal and reflects when someone's cognitive abilities have gotten to the point that the person can no longer independently do their typical daily activities (such as cooking meals and shopping). A lot of factors may contribute to dementia risk over time, and the most important causes of dementia are Alzheimer's disease and vascular disease. Both of these conditions can damage the brain over time.

Hearing loss and dementia — say what?

Over the past decade, research has shown that compared to those with normal hearing, people with hearing loss have a much higher risk of developing dementia.

Increasingly, researchers are beginning to understand why:

>> **Hearing loss can lead to social isolation and loneliness.** When people with hearing loss begin to feel uncomfortable in social situations, they often cut themselves off, which can lead to loneliness, loss of engagement in cognitively stimulating activities, and depression — all of which can increase a person's risk for dementia.

>> **Hearing loss overloads the circuitry of the brain.** With hearing loss, the brain is constantly having to work harder to process the degraded sounds coming from the ear. Scientists thinks that when this happens, the brain may have fewer resources (brain power!) to help preserve thinking and memory abilities.

>> **Hearing loss damages the brain.** Hearing loss leads to the brain being less stimulated with sound information, and this in turn appears to be linked with parts of the brain shrinking and atrophying faster from this chronic deprivation. As you can probably guess, an atrophying brain is not a good thing!

Scientists estimate, in fact, that hearing loss may be the biggest potentially treatable risk factor for dementia, accounting for more cases of dementia in the world than other risk factors such as high blood pressure, smoking, or low education.

Hearing aids to prevent dementia?

At this point, you may be scratching your head and asking something along the lines of "Uh . . . so are you telling me that people who have hearing loss are definitely going to get dementia?"

The answer to this, of course, is "No." Hearing loss may, however, increase your risk of dementia. Researchers can't predict the exact increase of risk for a given person.

The more important question, then, is whether strategies to address hearing loss such as hearing aids could actually help reduce someone's risk for dementia. Scientists think this *could* be the case, but they don't know yet for certain.

There is an ongoing randomized controlled trial that we're now leading in the United States funded by the National Institutes of Health, where people are randomly assigned to either get their hearing loss treated or not. We should know in a few years the results, telling us whether hearing loss treatment is linked to a reduced risk of cognitive decline and dementia.

In the meantime, the important thing to keep in mind is that addressing hearing loss with hearing aids and other strategies that are discussed later in this book come with virtually no health risks and could only have positive upsides for your ability to communicate and engage with others and possibly even benefits for your cognitive health. The degree to which these devices and strategies may reduce your risk for dementia remains to be determined, but there are clearly no downsides to addressing your hearing loss now.

2
Evaluating How You Hear

IN THIS PART . . .

Recognize signs of hearing loss and when to get tested.

Review how professionals assess and treat hearing loss and what to expect during a hearing test.

Understand how to make sense of your hearing test results and how it relates to your ability to hear sound.

Chapter **5**

Recognizing Hearing Loss

How would you characterize your hearing? It's a seemingly simple question, yet many don't know how to approach it.

Hearing loss is common. Really common. Over 38 million Americans have hearing loss in both ears while over 60 million Americans have hearing loss in at least one ear (that is nearly 1 in every 5 Americans!). Hearing loss becomes more common as we age. Nearly half of all adults over 60 years old have hearing loss.

Yet, most people don't recognize the extent of their own hearing loss and are unsure of the signs of hearing loss. Even those who may suspect their hearing is declining may be reluctant to acknowledge it for fear of being seen as "old."

But what kind of thinking is that? Hearing loss is just a fact of life. Whether we like it or not, most of us will develop some hearing loss. It's there, no getting around it. Being "old" depends on whether you let hearing loss hold you back from engaging with the world around you or whether you address it to ensure you thrive as you age.

This chapter helps you recognize whether you have hearing loss, discusses the merits of seeing a specialist and getting a hearing test, and counters the stigma surrounding hearing loss.

Missing the Signs of Hearing Loss

Many people aren't a very good judge of their own hearing. In fact, most people tend to believe their hearing is better than it actually is, according to research from our own team at Johns Hopkins University. Why are we such bad judges of our own ability to hear?

Barely noticeable changes

One answer is that hearing loss happens gradually and slowly over time. The snail-like pace at which our hearing declines may make it difficult to notice any changes. Early signs of hearing loss may be situational. We might miss a word here and there over dinner in a noisy restaurant or have trouble following a conversation with someone soft-spoken. It is easy to shrug off the seemingly isolated early incidents.

Everyone else is mumbling!

Hearing loss is about clarity not volume. Most people think of hearing loss as simply turning down the volume on a TV, which makes all sounds quieter. But hearing loss is more like turning down the volume on only specific frequencies or pitches of sound so while some sounds are quieter others are just as loud. For most people, hearing loss affects their ability to hear high frequencies (whistling or birds chirping) while leaving the ability to hear low frequencies (animal grunts or thunder) relatively untouched. Visit Chapter 2 for more information on how hearing works.

But not all sounds fit neatly into low or high frequencies. Speech has sounds from several frequencies. In fact, a single word can represent multiple frequencies. For example, the word "show" includes "sh" (high-frequency) and "ow" (low-frequency). With the most common types of hearing loss, the "sh" would be difficult to hear while "ow" would be perfectly audible. This results in a phenomenon where you would hear someone talking, but what they're saying isn't clear. This is why a common phrase among those with hearing loss is "I can hear you but you're mumbling!" Hearing some sounds but not others affects clarity, which isn't always something people think of when they think of hearing loss. Hence, sometimes it's hard to make that leap to suspecting hearing loss.

Compensating until you can't

Our brain plays a big role in making it tough to recognize hearing loss, especially when it first starts. Generally, our brains are great at their job of processing incoming information and can often still make sense of unclear speech. The brain does this by using contextual information like the general topic of conversation to fill in the blanks. This means that as we develop hearing loss, our brains initially do a pretty good job of making up for any hearing loss.

But compensating for hearing loss requires a lot of extra energy and effort from our brains. Over time, our hearing tends to worsen and our brain's ability to compensate lessens until it actually starts to slow down as well from the fatigue of keeping up with all the unclear sound. Take a look at Chapter 4 for more information on hearing loss and cognition.

Don't know what you're missing

Our brains are good at noticing new auditory information and ignoring common and mundane sound. Think about being in your own home versus visiting a place for the first time. In our own homes, we tend to ignore familiar sounds — the humming of appliances, creaking floorboards, or squeaking doors.

But in a new place, our brains are on high alert, and we notice every single new sound. The same concept goes for common environmental sounds when we aren't specifically listening for them: traffic noise from other cars while driving or chirping birds while walking through the park. When we aren't specifically listening for a sound, it often becomes forgotten background noise. This makes it difficult to realize what we miss when we have hearing loss.

Sussing Out Whether Your Hearing Has Declined

Given how difficult it is for us to judge our own hearing ability, consider having a conversation with those close to you to help you identify any hearing loss. Your hearing loss can impact them, too. In many situations, it is a spouse, child, companion, or other frequent communication partner who first detects signs of hearing loss — from little things like noticing you turn the TV up louder to feeling isolated from you because conversation has become more difficult. The perceptions of those around you is a great way to gauge your own hearing.

It is also often helpful to look for clues in how hearing may be affecting your day-to-day life. Consider, for example, any changes in your social activity, communication patterns, and regular activities to help identify any hearing loss. You may be subconsciously avoiding situations or even altering the way you engage with people because of difficulty hearing. Take a minute to ask yourself some of the following questions to get a better feel for whether you may have some hearing loss:

>> Are you asking others to repeat things more often? In follow-up, do you find others saying things like "Never mind, I'll tell you later" when you ask them to repeat something? This may be a sign that others have begun to notice your hearing difficulties.

>> Are you having trouble following conversations in meetings?

>> Do you find yourself believing many other people mumble too much?

>> Do you have difficulty hearing people when you aren't looking directly at them when they speak or when they turn away from you during conversation?

>> Have you felt embarrassed to contribute to conversations because you're unsure of the topic?

>> Do you feel excluded at dinner or other group conversations or unable to keep up?

>> Do you have any difficulty hearing small children? (People with hearing loss often find children's voices, which are higher pitched, difficult to understand.)

>> Do you turn up the volume on electronics such as the television?

>> Do you avoid talking on the telephone because it's fatiguing and hard to make out what the other person says?

>> Do others around you complain that the TV is too loud?

>> Do you find yourself avoiding restaurants or social gatherings more than you used to because they're too noisy?

>> Do you find yourself more tired than usual when engaging in conversation?

>> Are you avoiding activities you used to regularly participate in, such as attending concerts, plays, meetings, or religious services?

If you answered "yes" to any of these questions, it's a good idea to get your hearing tested. Read on to find out more.

Knowing When to Get Your Hearing Tested

We note earlier in this chapter that hearing loss is very common and that over half of all adults over the age of 60 experience hearing loss. It may be a good idea to schedule a hearing test if you notice any of the signs of hearing loss we outline earlier or when you turn 60 years of age, whichever comes first.

Screening, testing, and diagnostics

For this book, we're going to offer some definitions to help guide you while reading about assessing hearing. You may see the terms hearing screening or hearing testing thrown around and sometimes you'll see the term diagnostic hearing test versus self-guided hearing test. Here's what those mean:

» **Hearing screening** refers to any assessment or task that helps identify whether or not you likely have some hearing loss but offers little details. Hearing screenings vary in how they're performed and could be anything from whether you can hear someone whisper in your ear to a task where you have to identify numbers spoken in the presence of background noise.

» **Hearing testing** refers to pure-tone audiometry tests (see Chapter 7) that provides sufficient detail to describe your hearing in each ear using either the hearing number or categories like mild, moderate, severe, or profound.

» **Self-guided hearing testing** refers to hearing testing that is performed by you without the help of a professional, such as on a smartphone.

» **Diagnostic hearing testing** refers to a full battery of tests performed by a hearing professional, usually an audiologist, for the purpose of diagnosing hearing loss.

Establishing a baseline

A baseline hearing test simply refers to your first diagnostic hearing test, the results of which become the baseline or reference point for future hearing tests to keep track of any changes in hearing. The baseline test also helps hearing professionals create a custom plan for you based on patterns in changes in your hearing over time. Chapter 6 describes the details of a diagnostic hearing test in greater detail. We recommend establishing a baseline as soon as you suspect hearing loss or at least by the time you turn 60, even if you're not particularly concerned with your hearing at the moment.

Making the appointment

Here are the details you need to know to make an appointment:

» Insurance, including Medicare, usually covers at least one diagnostic hearing test a year when ordered by a physician (check with your provider when in doubt).

» An audiologist (see Chapter 6) will usually perform the diagnostic hearing test.

>> Request a referral from your primary care provider (if required by your insurance company).

>> Search online for a local audiologist near you that accepts your insurance or use websites like HearingTracker.com, which maintains a directory of audiologists from across the country with patient reviews.

TIP

Curious to do some testing on your own hearing? Try one of numerous smartphone- or web-based hearing tests and screeners such as Mimi Hearing or SonicCloud, which are free and can be found in your smartphone app store, or the AARP at-home hearing screener found at nationalhearingtest.org (free for AARP members!).

Getting the results

After a diagnostic hearing test, the audiologist will go over the results with you. This professional can describe your hearing patterns and give you an idea of your overall hearing with terms like normal, mild, or moderate hearing loss. Always request a copy of the results for your own record! Chapter 7 goes over how to read the results from a diagnostic hearing test in full detail.

Because you have this book, you're well equipped to ask for extra details. We recommend asking for your hearing number (also known as the four-frequency pure-tone average) in addition to your category of hearing. We explain in Chapter 7 how you can calculate the hearing number on your own.

TECHNICAL STUFF

Your *hearing number* indicates how loud speech sounds have to be for you to hear them. The number ranges from approximately 0 dB (really soft) to 100 dB (really loud) so the lower your hearing number is, the better your hearing. The typical cutoff point used to classify someone as having a clinically significant hearing loss is 25.

One of the reasons we recommend a baseline diagnostic hearing test early on is to have an anchor point for determining just how much your hearing changes. The hearing number can help show just how much change you experience over time compared to just being told that you have a mild or moderate hearing loss.

Consider the following scenario: You get your hearing tested when you're 50 years old and have a hearing number of 5, which is well within the "normal" hearing range. Then you get your hearing tested when you're 65 and your hearing number is 34, which is within the "mild" hearing loss range. That's a huge change in your hearing number, and any hearing professional would recommend addressing it and monitoring you closely via annual hearing tests. But without that baseline, you might feel like the "mild" hearing loss label means it's no big deal and shrug it off for the time being. Having a grasp of your own change in hearing with the rise in the hearing number (rather than just knowing you have a "normal" or "mild" hearing loss) is key to understanding what's going on with your hearing and what you can do about it.

TIP

If you have a smartphone, you can obtain your hearing number yourself without even needing to see an audiologist. Go to www.hearingnumber.org to learn more.

Getting regular hearing checkups

After establishing your baseline hearing results, it's a good idea to schedule a follow-up hearing test every year or every two years with a professional, such as an audiologist, or create a plan to regularly monitor your hearing via various self-guided hearing test methods (see Chapter 6 for more information). Even if your baseline hearing test suggests no sign of hearing loss, your hearing can change as you age.

REMEMBER

Getting hearing tests regularly can help you stay in front of any changes in hearing and act early if you develop hearing loss. Acting early does not have to mean pursuing hearing aids right away (although that may be a good option if you need them — see Chapter 9). Acting early could be adopting some simple strategies at first, including being cognizant of using noise protection to preserve hearing, using communication techniques, or learning to use other everyday technologies for difficult listening situations (see Chapter 8 for these strategies). Importantly, acting early sets you on the right path to addressing hearing loss and pursuing various incremental hearing care options as needed.

WARNING

The longer you wait to begin addressing your hearing loss, the more difficult it may be to eventually adapt to using various communication strategies and hearing technologies. In particular, hearing aids do amazing things, but they are not a panacea that restores your hearing to normal (see Chapter 19 for other common myths and misunderstandings about hearing loss). It takes time to get used to using hearing aids and other technologies like a cochlear implant and the longer you live with unaddressed hearing loss, the harder it is to adjust later to using these hearing technologies.

Knowing when you should get tested immediately

The vast majority of hearing loss is not considered urgent or an emergency requiring same-day testing and treatment. But if you experience a sudden change in hearing, then it's time to call the ear, nose, and throat (ENT) doctor immediately and schedule a comprehensive hearing exam. Trauma to the ear and dizziness or vertigo accompanied with a change in hearing and/or tinnitus also warrants contacting an ENT quickly. Some sudden hearing losses can be corrected via medical treatment if addressed in a timely fashion. Chapter 13 covers medically related hearing loss in deeper detail.

Shrugging Off the Stigma of Hearing Loss

Society's view of hearing loss is complicated and has a long history. Unfortunately, over the years, discrimination, ableism, and ageism have painted hearing loss in a very negative light. Think of movies and TV that characterize people with hearing loss and hearing aids as frail older adults, reinforcing a damaging stereotype. Fortunately, we are well beyond a deep negative view of hearing loss as a society, but some stigma of hearing loss still exists.

Much of the persistent stigma around hearing loss is that many associate it with being old (despite the fact that hearing diminishes slowly over our entire lifetime). What better way to combat the negative stigma of being old than to identify hearing loss early and improve your hearing so that you can continue to participate in the world around you?

TOP THREE REASONS NOT TO LET STIGMA GET IN YOUR WAY OF HEARING CARE

- **Staying connected with friends and family** is a vital part of life. While it may not seem like it at times, humans are social creatures. Talking to one another to share stories and opinions is a key part of how we connect. Hearing loss can be isolating by cutting you off from those conversations. By addressing your hearing loss, you can ensure you're able to engage with your loved ones.

- **Engaging in work, hobbies, and activities** is a part of our identity. Performing the activities in life that we enjoy reduces stress and improves quality of life. Hearing loss can be a barrier to performing our job duties, such as making calls and participating in meetings, and prevent us from participating in our favorite activities like listening to music or attending the theater. By not addressing hearing loss, you can miss out on these important activities.

- **Keeping your mind sharp** is possible by addressing your hearing loss. Making sense of sound with hearing loss takes a lot of effort and can wear you down. Addressing hearing loss can reduce fatigue and help you engage in activities and connect with others. The result is that addressing your hearing loss could help you maintain cognitive vitality.

Caring about your hearing above what other people think

First, let's get this out of the way: Who cares what anyone else thinks? Are we right? Your needs and ability to live a joyful life by acknowledging and addressing your hearing loss via any combination of hearing care options are your own business. Comparing yourself to others and letting their judgment of you hamper your desired well-being is no way to live.

Along these lines, we often hear, "Well, my friend Joe Anybody has hearing loss and doesn't do anything about it, so why should I?" The answer to this is simple: You're not Joe Anybody. We all have our own unique pattern of hearing and, with it, our own unique hearing needs. There is no point comparing your needs to others; no two hearing loss experiences are the same. Addressing your hearing loss can improve your life: your relationships, your cognitive health, your physical health, your balance, and so much more. Consider the detrimental outcomes of dementia, loneliness, and falls that researchers have all found linked with hearing loss and that we discuss in Chapter 4. Don't let what other people think stand in the way of living a fuller life.

It's okay to wear hearing aids

In the clinic, we often hear something along the lines of "but won't hearing aids make me look old?" We often answer this question with "Well, what would make someone look older? An inability to participate in conversation and asking people to repeat themselves or actively engaging in discussion and maintaining strong social connections?" We say this playfully, of course, but the question is valid and the response has merit.

When confronted with pushback from stigma, we focus on the benefit of addressing hearing loss to meet our patients' personal goals. Whether that is hearing a loved one whisper to them or ensuring they don't miss a beat during work meetings. To us, the stigma associated with hearing aids is counterintuitive. If addressing hearing loss can help you live a happy and fulfilling life, then hearing aids are decidedly not making you look "old." By pursuing hearing care that meets your needs and makes you a vital member of your world, you're living the life you want to live, staying socially connected and cognitively active, and engaging with the world around you.

TODAY'S TRENDS FIGHT THE STIGMA

Hearing loss is common and it's going to be even more common in the future because people are living longer. In fact, the 85+ years of age group is the fastest growing demographic in the United States. Projections from Johns Hopkins University show the number of Americans living with hearing loss will double in the next 40 years. You're not alone.

Hearing aids and other hearing technology are quickly becoming fashion statements of vibrant, tech savvy individuals. Ear level technology such as earbuds or Bluetooth devices are ubiquitous in society. Companies such as Apple and Bose are increasingly focusing on the design and look of their products in addition to the sound quality. Modern hearing aids are no different; they're sleek and discrete. Some hearing aids are even moving towards designs that make them indistinguishable from earbuds.

Hearing aids are simply becoming more common. A perfect storm for increased uptake in hearing aids has occurred at the time of this book. Note the following:

- New research on links between hearing loss and healthy aging to increase awareness of the importance of hearing loss.
- Big advances in digital hearing aid technology to improve sound quality.
- The introduction of over-the-counter (OTC) hearing aids that is driving consumer tech companies to create hearing aids and making them often indistinguishable from other consumer earbuds. This opening of the market to OTC hearing aids will also vastly improve accessibility and affordability.

The result is a rise in hearing aid use. It's hard to stigmatize something when it's so common.

The stigma is fading

First, we like to believe that society is moving beyond ableism and ageism and dropping the irrational stigma associated with hearing loss. Second, as more and more adults acknowledge and address hearing loss, the stigma will rapidly fade.

At the writing of this book, only 20 percent of Americans with hearing loss own and use hearing aids. While not every single person with hearing loss would immediately benefit from hearing aids, it is much higher than 20 percent. Chapter 9 provides some details on barriers to hearing aid adoption. But use of hearing aids seems to be on the upswing. Hearing aid ownership increased nearly 22 percent among Medicare beneficiaries in the United States from 2008 to 2018, according to data from Johns Hopkins University. Increased uptake will destigmatize hearing aids. Consider: If even half of the adults over 60 who have hearing loss used hearing aids, then a quarter of all adults over 60 years would use hearing aids. It's hard to stigmatize something when it is that pervasive in society. Think of eyeglasses. Would you think poorly of someone just because they used corrective lenses?

New over-the-counter (OTC) hearing aids may fundamentally change the face of hearing care and further add to the decline in stigma. Chapter 9 covers these new products for adults with mild and moderate hearing loss, just approved by the U.S. Food and Drug Administration. We expect that these new OTC hearing aids will improve accessibility and affordability of devices and spur innovation to create some exciting and perhaps more stylish hearing device options.

Chapter **6**

Seeing a Hearing Loss Professional and Getting Tested

I f you suspect you might have hearing loss, you may be eager to jump right to hearing care options such as the newly available over-the-counter hearing aids. Well, let's put the brakes on for a minute.

A good first step is to get a diagnostic hearing test by a professional to find out what's going on. You may immediately think, *Why bother with a professional and a test if I already know I have trouble with my hearing?* This is a totally reasonable question.

Here's why: The details a professional will reveal are key! That diagnostic hearing test can be a critical step before jumping right into hearing care options. The assessment is vital to fully describing the degree and nature of your hearing loss and ruling out any medical conditions that could play a role. Think of hearing like fingerprints — everyone has their own unique patterns. With your distinctive hearing fully characterized, those results can help determine what hearing care options are best for you. And, should you obtain hearing aids, the professionals will have the information needed to create custom programs to address your unique hearing (more on that in Chapter 9).

But where do you start with getting a diagnostic hearing test and what should you expect? It can be intimidating to start a new hearing journey. Fortunately, we're here to break it down for you. In this chapter, you find out about the hearing professionals and what each specializes in. Then we cover the various tests they perform and what the results tell you about your hearing.

"A journey of a thousand miles begins with a single step." Let's take that first step on your hearing journey and explore seeing a hearing professional to get your hearing assessed.

Getting to Know the Hearing Care Team

Did you know there are several different fields that address hearing loss? We tend to think there's just one sort of "hearing expert" or "hearing doctor," but really three distinct specialists each play a unique role. In the following sections, we explain who these folks are and what they do so you can determine who you need on your team.

REMEMBER

It is very common to see more than one professional to meet your unique hearing needs.

WARNING

Buyer beware. When selecting a professional for a hearing test, remember that some things are too good to be true. Some companies advertising "Free Hearing Tests" may be more interested in selling a hearing aid than providing a hearing test.

Audiologist: Assessing and addressing hearing loss

One of this book's authors, Dr. Nicholas Reed, is an audiologist. These professionals identify, diagnose, and manage hearing loss with comprehensive hearing testing and best-practice hearing care that includes a combination of technologic and counseling techniques (see Chapter 9 for more information on hearing care).

Audiologists are not physicians or medical doctors; rather, they hold doctorates and specialize in hearing and *vestibular* (an aspect of balance) science. Audiologists perform comprehensive hearing test batteries, review the results with their patients, and make recommendations for next steps. They also specialize in addressing hearing loss via several options, including technology recommendations, hearing aid or cochlear implant fitting, counseling and training on communication strategies for people with hearing loss, and helping to navigate the over-the-counter hearing device market. Audiologists often work side by side with ear, nose, and throat doctors, also called *otolaryngologists,* to provide the right combination of medical (otolaryngology) and rehabilitative (audiology) hearing care.

When seeking an audiologist, look for certifications that indicate a high level of continuous post-graduate training such as American Board of Audiology (ABA) certification from the American Academy of Audiology or the Certificate of Clinical Competence in Audiology (CCC-A) from the American Speech-Language-Hearing Association.

Otolaryngologist: Comprehensive medical care for the ear

An otolaryngologist — like the other author of this book, Dr. Frank Lin — is responsible for the medical assessment of the auditory system. Otolaryngologists are physicians who specialize in the ears, nose, and throat — hence, they're often referred to as ENTs for short. These doctors undergo over a decade of training between medical school, residency, and fellowships. Dr. Lin spends a significant portion of his time talking to patients about their hearing loss, treating ear disease, and performing ear surgeries.

While the otolaryngologist doesn't actually perform the hearing test (that's usually done by an audiologist; see the previous section), the otolaryngologist plays a comprehensive role in putting your hearing and ear health into the context of your overall medical health and creating a treatment plan. During your appointment, the otolaryngologist will review your medical history; go over the results of the hearing test; examine your ear, nose, and throat; and review and order other tests as needed, such as radiologic imaging.

After reviewing everything, the otolaryngologist will give a formal diagnosis of your type of hearing loss or other medical conditions (if applicable), discuss the potential origins of your hearing loss, and explore your options to medically correct certain types of hearing losses, such as conductive hearing loss (see Chapter 13), via surgery. Otolaryngologists also perform the surgeries for special hearing devices such as cochlear implants for severe hearing loss. We talk about that more in Chapter 13.

Look for otolaryngologists who are certified by the American Board of Otolaryngology-Head & Neck Surgery, indicating they have passed a specialized exam and meet a higher standard of knowledge. If possible, you can also look for an otolaryngologist who specifically specializes in otology or neurotology. These specialized ENTs (also called otologists or neurotologists) have had further advanced fellowship training after residency specifically in the ear.

Hearing instrument specialist: Focusing on the hearing aid

Hearing instrument specialists play a highly specialized role in hearing care. They are licensed to sell and dispense hearing aids by the state in which they do business. Unlike audiologists and otolaryngologists, hearing instrument specialists do not have national education requirements. Instead, each state sets its own requirements for licensure; usually the core requirement is passing a state-administered exam. These requirements can vary greatly from state to state. In many rural areas, hearing instrument specialists are the only place to get a hearing test as there is a dearth of otolaryngologists and audiologists in the United States.

When it comes to assessing hearing loss, hearing instrument specialists can and do perform some basic parts of a hearing tests for the purpose of selecting and fitting a hearing aid. They cannot, however, bill an insurance provider for the exam or offer a formal interpretation of the results or a diagnosis of hearing loss. Because their scope is narrow, these specialists may perform only a few hearing tests rather than a comprehensive battery of tests to assess the auditory system. Hearing aids are where hearing instrument specialists shine. They provide a range of hearing aid services, including selection, fitting, and maintenance.

The most important team member: You!

That's right. You're a key member of the team. Hearing loss is not a short-term condition with a quick fix. It is considered a long-term chronic condition that requires repeated assessments over time to monitor hearing and make continuous adjustments in your hearing care plan to meet any changes in hearing or lifestyle. Whether you like it or not, you play a role as the manager who keeps track of past history, monitors your hearing, maintains any hearing devices, and stays alert to any changes that may require the attention of a professional.

TIP

A key role that you play is preparing for your visits with hearing professionals. A great way to prepare for a diagnostic hearing test visit is to think about answers to the hearing history questions you see in the next section of this chapter. The more information you give a hearing professional, the better they can meet your needs.

Preparing for the Assessment

Once you know the types of professionals, it's time to schedule an appointment. To have a diagnostic hearing test performed, look for your local audiologist's office. Here are some quick tips when scheduling an appointment:

>> Most insurance covers a hearing exam at least once a year, but check with your insurer to see if you need a physician's referral.

>> Call your insurance carrier or visit its website to see which audiologists in your area are in-network.

>> Ask your primary care doctor for a referral to an audiologist (if needed).

>> Search online for local audiologists or use directories like the American Academy of Audiology.

>> Ask friends or your local Hearing Loss Association of America chapter for recommendations.

WARNING

If you're scheduling an appointment for a sudden change in your hearing, pain, dizziness, vertigo, or any active drainage from your ear, start with an otolaryngologist or check with your primary care doctor first.

TIP

It can be difficult to know where to start when it comes to finding a hearing professional. Aside from some of the certifications we've mentioned in this chapter, how do you know if the professional is "good"? It can be extremely helpful to talk to your peers about their experiences with local hearing professionals and use websites like www.hearingtracker.com that let the public comment on professionals and share their experiences.

It all starts with history

Your initial hearing appointment — whether with an audiologist, ENT, or hearing instrument specialist — should always include a comprehensive history, ideally at the beginning of the appointment. These questions can guide what hearing tests are selected, determine how the hearing tests are performed, and lead to other test recommendations and treatment options. Expect questions such as the following:

>> Have you had previous noise exposure from your occupation, leisure activities, or firearm use?

>> Do you have a history of ear infections or surgeries?

>> Do you have any trouble understanding people talking such as on a phone, in quiet settings, or in noisy settings like a restaurant?

>> Do you have any trouble understanding speech or following conversations in your primary language on television or radio?

>> Do you have a preferred listening ear?

>> When did your hearing problem start? Was it gradual or sudden?

>> What activities does your lifestyle entail?

TIP

Any hearing assessment visit that doesn't include your hearing history with questions like those in the preceding list is missing out on the most important factor: your experience and perception. It could be a sign of a practitioner who's more interested in selling a hearing aid than providing best-practice hearing care.

To know the ear is to see the ear

At hearing care visits, a professional — whether audiologist, ENT, or hearing instrument specialist — will want to physically examine your ear. The medical term for this is *otoscopy*. During otoscopy, the hearing professional will insert the tip of an *otoscope* (see Figure 6-1), an instrument for looking in the ear, into your ear canal. The professional is looking for the general health and anatomical shape of the ear canal and eardrum (see Chapter 2 for details on ear anatomy), presence of excessive earwax, and any foreign bodies or debris in the ear canal. This helps inform what may be contributing to any hearing loss and is crucial to make sure it is safe to put an earphone in your ears for the tests that will follow.

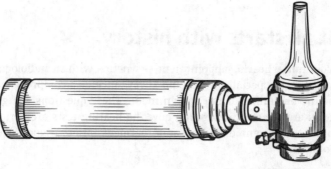

FIGURE 6-1:
An otoscope, which is used to look into the ear.

Source: John Wiley & Sons, Inc.

Knowing What to Expect during the First Part of the Diagnostic Hearing Test

Once a history is complete and the hearing professional has looked in your ears, it's time for the actual hearing tests. The entire diagnostic hearing test consists of several different tests, from responding to tones or beeps to repeating back words. Most professionals begin with a pure-tone hearing test.

Picking up on pure-tones: "Listen for the beeps"

The pure-tone hearing test is the foundation of the diagnostic hearing test battery. It uses something called *pure-tones* (we know, we know, no one has ever accused hearing care of being creative with their names). Pure-tones are signals at a single frequency; for example, just 500 Hz or just 1,000 Hz (Hz stands for hertz; check out Chapter 2 for more information). Most hearing tests assess 250, 500, 1,000, 2,000, 4,000, and 8,000 Hz at minimum; sometimes other frequencies such as 3,000 Hz and 6,000 Hz are included.

We rarely hear pure-tones in our everyday listening environments. Speech, for example, is a much more complex auditory signal with thousands of overlapping pure-tones. We like to think of pure-tones as single, individual keys on a piano. Alone, they aren't very interesting, but once we put them together, well, that's when the magic happens.

You've got to be thinking "Nick and Frank, you make no sense; if we rarely hear pure-tones, why do we use them for testing?" Good point. The reason we begin with the testing of pure-tones is because pure-tones help us identify exactly where you might have trouble hearing sound and provide a clearer picture for where to give you a boost with hearing aids or amplification. Conversely, if we were to rely only on speech testing, we couldn't easily distinguish exactly where you have trouble hearing because speech spreads across many frequencies (approximately 500 to 4000 Hz).

REMEMBER

Hearing loss does not occur equally across all frequencies or pitches. It often affects high-frequencies or pitches.

The test usually takes place in a sound booth (see Figure 6-2) with thick walls to prevent outside noise from interfering with the test. Some modern equipment, however, allows for hearing assessments outside of a sound booth.

Once seated in the booth, you may suddenly notice wires everywhere. *What could require that many wires?* The answer is an audiometer, a highly specialized piece of equipment that is calibrated to produce precise sounds that measure your hearing ability. We measure hearing in several different ways, some of which require different headsets (and accompanying wires!). The hearing professional will either fit you with over-the-ear headphones or insert earphones for testing.

Once situated, you will be instructed to sit quietly and wait until you hear beeps or tones. Once you hear a beep, you'll let the professional know by either pressing a button or raising your hand. The beeps will get softer and softer until you no longer hear them. It's important that you respond even if you *think* you hear the

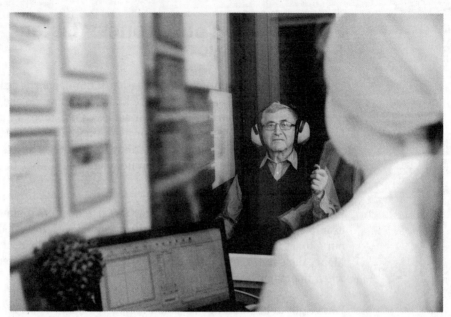

Source: John Wiley & Sons, Inc.

FIGURE 6-2:
Taking a hearing
test in a booth.

beep. The lowest volume you can respond to repeatedly is then marked as your threshold for that frequency. This process will occur across all frequencies tested for each ear.

TIP

Try out a pure-tone hearing test yourself! Look for the free Mimi or SonicCloud hearing test apps in your smartphone's app store or go to www.hearingnumber. org to learn about ways to take a pure-tone hearing test yourself with a smartphone.

Testing your hearing with air and bone conduction

In addition to the pure-tone tests at several frequencies in each ear (see the preceding section), you'll also complete pure-tone tests with two different modalities: air conduction, which assesses the entire auditory system, and bone-conduction, which isolates the response from the cochlea.

Assessing the entire auditory system

The auditory system is made up of multiple areas, including an outer, middle, and inner ear. In Chapter 2, we discuss how sound gets from the environment around you all the way to your brain.

To assess the entire auditory system, we use either earphones or over-the-head headphones (see Figure 6-3). Sound leaves the speakers in the earphones or headphones to enter air in the ear canal and then travels across the eardrum, the middle ear space, and into the cochlea. This process is called *air conduction* because the sound is being conducted through the air in your ear (see Figure 6-4).

Bypassing the outer and middle ear

Did you know sound can travel through the bones in our body via vibrations? You may not have realized it, but we bet you've experienced this sensation your entire life. Think about chewing something crunchy, like potato chips, with your mouth closed; it can sound as loud as a tractor, right? But does it sound as loud to your friend sitting across the table? The answer is no. The sound vibrations from chewing in your mouth travel along the bones and directly stimulate the cochlea (inner ear), while those same vibrations have to travel through air to reach another person's ear. Because bone is denser than air, it is a better conductor of sound. We call this phenomenon *bone conduction*.

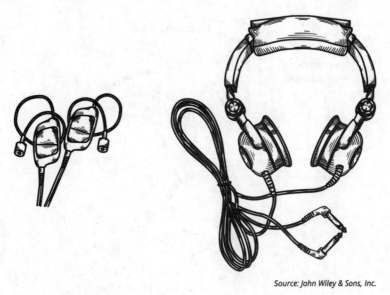

FIGURE 6-3:
Earphones (left) and over-the-ear headphones (right).

Source: John Wiley & Sons, Inc.

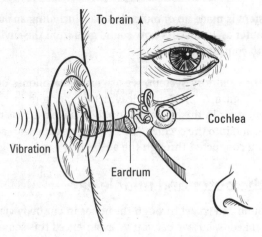

Air conduction

To brain

Cochlea

Vibration

Eardrum

FIGURE 6-4:
Air conduction.

Source: John Wiley & Sons, Inc.

A device called a *bone oscillator* is used to perform bone conduction pure-tone hearing tests. The bone oscillator creates vibrations to produce pure-tone signals. It usually sits behind the ear on an area referred to as the mastoid or directly on the center of the forehead, held snuggly in place by a fitted band (see Figure 6-5).

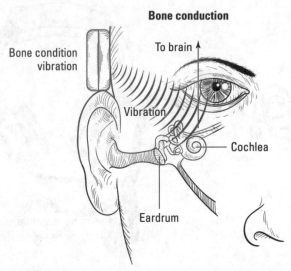

Bone conduction

Bone condition vibration

To brain

Vibration

Cochlea

Eardrum

FIGURE 6-5:
Bone conduction.

Source: John Wiley & Sons, Inc.

Why assess both air and bone conduction?

By assessing hearing with both air and bone conduction, the hearing professional can determine what area is contributing to any hearing loss as well as the type of hearing loss (more on the types of hearing loss in Chapter 7). For example, if a person has good hearing with bone conduction but poorer hearing with air conduction, then something is blocking that sound from getting into the cochlear, such as fluid in the ear or an ear canal completely full of wax.

Checking Out Other Hearing Assessment Measures

In addition to the pure-tone hearing testing and air and bone conduction, many other assessments can help provide a comprehensive assessment of the entire auditory system.

Testing whether sound is getting to the middle and inner ears

To help diagnose the cause of hearing problems, professionals may include one or two tests that provide insight into how the middle ear space is functioning and transmitting sound to the cochlea. This type of testing is known as *immittance testing.* To complete immittance tests, a small earpiece is inserted into the ear canal to create an airtight seal, which allows the earpiece to measure any pressure changes from movement of the eardrum.

The most common immittance test is called *tympanometry,* which tests the mobility of the eardrum by gently moving the air between the earpiece and the eardrum. The test can assess if the eardrum is too stiff or too loose, which may suggest an issue in the middle ear space. This test also checks the volume of space in the ear canal; abnormally large volume may suggest a hole in the eardrum.

Another common test is called *acoustic reflex testing.* During this test, a loud tone is produced. In response to that tone, a muscle in the middle ear tenses up and causes all the small bones in the ear (*ossicles*) to tighten up. Professionals use this test to get an idea of the integrity of the entire auditory system because that loud tone had to make its way all the way through the outer, middle, and inner ear to the brain and then trigger the brain to send a signal back to the muscle.

TECHNICAL STUFF

Wait ... what? Did you read that right? The brain sends a signal back to the muscle in the ear? Yes! Our brain is pretty amazing and responds rapidly to various inputs, including sound. In a way, the acoustic reflex is just like your knee jerk reflex.

Measuring your speech understanding

Up to this point, we've discussed tests that involve responding to simple beeps and tones or looking at how the ear functions and the eardrum moves. These are essential for understanding how the outer, middle, and inner ear detect sound. Sometimes we refer to these as peripheral hearing assessments, meaning that they only represent parts of the auditory system (the outer, middle, and inner ear) that capture and encode sound before the sound is sent to the central auditory system (the brain), where it is processed for understanding.

But our patients are most concerned with understanding and processing speech, not detecting tones. Speech understanding is a more complex process that involves both the ear and the brain. So now we turn our attention to assessments that measure processing of sound such as speech understanding.

Words, sentences, and phrases, oh my!

During a diagnostic hearing test, you may complete several different tests that include the use of words, sentences, and phrases.

Speech reception testing involves the hearing professional either saying or playing prerecorded two-syllable words through the earphones or headphones and asking you to repeat the words back. The words will become sequentially softer and softer in volume and even become so soft they are inaudible. (When you're taking these tests, always guess! More often than not, your first guess is correct, but many people don't trust themselves and give up before they've really reached their lowest threshold.) The lowest level at which a patient can correctly repeat back a word is called the *speech reception threshold* and provides information on detecting speech.

The speech reception threshold should match up neatly with the averaged thresholds of certain frequencies from the pure-tone testing. Specifically, the pure-tone average refers to the average of pure-tone thresholds at 500, 1,000, 2,000, and 4,000 Hz. These four frequencies represent the most important region for speech understanding, and the average threshold will be close to where an individual can detect speech. It serves as a reliability check to build confidence in the collective results of the entire hearing test.

TECHNICAL STUFF

For adults who are nonverbal and can't repeat back words, hearing professionals use a speech awareness threshold as opposed to the speech reception threshold. The speech awareness threshold does not require the patient to repeat the word, just to indicate whether they are aware of speech sound being produced.

Word recognition testing involves the hearing professional either saying or playing prerecorded one-syllable words at a steady, loud but comfortable level that should be easy for the patient to hear based off the pure-tone testing already completed. The patient is asked to repeat back the words. The number of words presented can range from 10 to 50. The final word recognition score is the percent repeated correctly. This test moves beyond detecting sound and focuses on how well you can process sound when played at a level that should be audible for you.

A last area of speech testing, *sentence understanding* can be any number of tests that all involve different types of sentences or phrases. The choice of test is at the discretion of the hearing professional. Regardless of the test, sentence understanding is generally presented at a comfortable listening level and, like the word recognition score, provides information on processing speech.

REMEMBER

An interesting tidbit is that understanding a sentence is an easier task than understanding a single word. This is because sentences put together several words that give contextual information to help us decipher everything. For example, you may have trouble hearing the word "cat" and confuse it for the word "sat" when those words are presented without context. But if someone says the sentence, "Please feed the . . .," the extra contextual information helps you decide they're likely saying "cat" and not "sat."

WARNING

A poor word recognition score or sentence understanding score indicates that making sound louder alone may not be enough because even at loud but comfortable amplified levels of sound, you still had trouble understanding speech. This could mean hearing aids aren't going to be your best option and could trigger a referral for cochlear implants (see Chapter 13). Your hearing care professional will give you their clinical insights and recommendations for further testing or treatment options.

With or without noise?

Life is noisy. It only makes sense that some tests are performed in the presence of background noise to assess how we hear in a situation closer to everyday life.

Speech in noise tests, as they're called, present either single words or sentences in the presence of background noise. The background noise may be either static noise or multi-talker babble that sounds rather like a restaurant full of conversations occurring all at once. The patient is asked to repeat back the words or sentences. The difficulty of the test depends on how close the words or speech (the signal) are to the background noise in volume. For example, speech presented at 70 decibels with 50-decibel background noise (relatively clear conversation in setting with mild background noise) is easier to make out than a signal presented at 70 decibels with 65-decibel background noise (tough to understand conversation where the noise is just as loud as the talkers — like a busy restaurant that is also playing the music way too loud). This test determines the level at which your brain can no longer focus or make out the sound you want to hear from competing background noise.

Understanding speech in noise is a demanding task that puts pressure on the brain to disentangle the signal of interest from the competing background noise. Many hearing care professionals use speech in noise assessments as a powerful counseling tool to help set expectations for patients when they're wearing hearing aids in difficult listening environments with lots of background noise.

Evaluating how the brain reacts to sound

A hearing test that requires no input from the patient is a truly objective test. These are incredibly valuable in healthcare. The most commonly used objective tests are *otoacoustic emissions* and the *auditory brainstem response*. These tests are used sparingly in adults for hearing assessments, however, and are much more common in infants and children who wouldn't be able to respond reliably to indicate that they heard a tone. You may encounter these tests, so here's a quick overview of what to expect.

Back in Chapter 2, we discuss those tiny hair cells in the inner ear. An amazing thing about those hair cells is that when they detect and encode a signal to be sent to the brain, that process creates a sound that we can measure all the way from the ear canal. We refer to that sound as *otoacoustic emissions.* To perform the otoacoustic emissions test, a professional will place a small earpiece in the ear, and you'll hear some tones and beeps. Just sit still and wait. After only a minute or two, the test is over. That's it! The otoacoustic emissions test is a screener that will give a general indication of whether you have some hearing loss or not.

During the *auditory brainstem response test*, small electrodes are placed around a patient's head. Then tones are played in the patient's ear. Again, you don't need to do anything but sit still and wait for the test to finish (you can even sleep!). The electrodes pick up the neurologic signal produced in the cochlea as it moves to the brain. This measurement of the brain's reaction to sound can be used to understand both how a person's auditory system detects tones and whether the auditory pathways to the brain are functioning normally.

Testing when sound is clear but difficult to understand

Other specialized tests of sound processing in the brain include

>> Tasks where the patient is presented with different words or phrases to each ear at the same time

>> Tasks where the patient is asked to localize the direction a sound came from

>> Tasks that involve understanding and deciphering speech that is purposefully degraded, speeded up, or slowed down

>> Tasks where the patient is asked to detect gaps or pauses in continuously presented noise or indicate patterns of tones presented in short and long bursts

These tests are generally considered only for patients suspected of having an auditory processing disorder. This is a relatively rare condition diagnosed mainly in children (but occasionally in adults), where the brain has more difficulty with decoding and processing sound signals despite a normal peripheral hearing system (cochlea). An auditory processing disorder in adults usually is related to other medical conditions such as problems with concentrating or other thinking and memory problems.

REMEMBER

It is important to note that the vast majority of auditory processing disorder assessments and diagnoses are done in children.

One and Done or a Regular Occurrence?

At the end of the appointment, the hearing professional will go over the results. This is a great time to ask questions and discuss any next steps. One of those next steps should be thinking about when to get another test.

TIP

Request a copy of your hearing test results to keep for your own records and to share with other professionals in the future!

If you go on to get prescription hearing aids, you'll schedule periodic hearing tests to customize the hearing aids to your unique hearing pattern. Even when using over-the-counter hearing aids, regular hearing testing can help either in customizing the device at home or determining when it's time to change to a different level of device. The hearing results can even help guide the use of different communication techniques (see Chapter 8) to address hearing loss.

No matter where you are in the hearing care process, it is important to plan for annual or biannual comprehensive diagnostic hearing tests. Regular assessments can monitor your hearing and help you recognize when it is time to act. Engaging in hearing care early is important, because waiting too long can make it hard to adjust to devices in the future. Moreover, as we discuss in Chapter 4, mounting evidence points to the association between unaddressed hearing loss and social isolation, loneliness, depression, cognitive decline, and more. As with any chronic medical condition, acting early rather than waiting until later is key to minimizing the impact of the condition on your life.

Chapter **7**

Making Sense of Your Hearing Test Results

I f you're anything like us, when you see your doctor, you try to focus on every-thing said during the appointment but when you walk out, *poof!*, it's like you retained only half the conversation and all you're left with is a report full of medical jargon that you can barely decipher. So, what do you do now?

That's where this chapter comes in. Maybe you've had a diagnostic hearing test with a professional and reviewed the results but can't remember what your hear-ing care professional told you. Or, alternatively, you've completed a self-guided hearing test using an app and need a little help figuring out what the results actu-ally mean. Or you're ready to get tested and want to be prepared. Well, we're here to help!

In this chapter, we go over the results from a hearing test and what they mean to you. We also introduce a newer, easier way to describe hearing via the hearing number. And we touch on what your test results mean for your next step in your hearing care journey.

REMEMBER

In this book, the term *hearing test* refers to pure-tone audiometry, which involves finding the softest tone you can hear at various pitches or frequencies. A *diagnostic hearing test* refers to when a professional conducts the audiometric testing often in conjunction with additional tests to get a complete picture of the status of your hearing. A *self-guided hearing test* is when you complete pure-tone audiometry on your own (generally with a smartphone).

Understanding the Importance of Reading Results

Following a diagnostic hearing test, the hearing care professional should review the results with you and provide recommendations. But usually this occurs for only a few minutes at the end of the appointment. Everything the professional covered doesn't always stick or you think of follow-up questions later.

TIP

You should always ask for a copy of your test results for your records. Sometimes this comes with a summary from the hearing professional, but often it's just a copy of a graph called the *audiogram* (more on that in the upcoming section "Audiogram 101") without any orientation or direction on how to read it.

Alternatively, there are an increasing number of self-guided hearing tests that provide pure-tone audiometry results that you can do on a smartphone app, such as Mimi or SonicCloud. While many apps do a thorough job of explaining the results, some may offer little guidance (see the upcoming section "How to get your hearing number").

As the era of over-the-counter hearing aids (see Chapter 10) arrives where many individuals will select and adjust hearing aids without the need to go through a professional, we think it's important you're equipped with the right knowledge to make sense of your test results. Being able to interpret the results can help you make the right decision when selecting and adjusting an over-the-counter hearing aid or knowing when to see a professional for help and guidance.

Introducing the Audiogram: What Does That Graph Mean?

REMEMBER

The most common method of showing test results is the audiogram, a graphical representation of the *hearing thresholds* obtained during the hearing test. The hearing thresholds are the softest level at which you can reliably detect or hear tones of different pitches during a hearing test.

Hearing thresholds can be measured using both air and bone conduction (see Chapter 6) to assess how different aspects of the auditory system are functioning. But for interpreting the results, we focus on the air-conduction thresholds only. This test is the most meaningful result for most people as these results directly indicate how much sound is getting from the environment into your ear and then to your brain. In other words, it tells you about sounds you can and cannot hear.

Audiogram 101

Figure 7-1 shows a standard audiogram graph with several images. At first glance, it's kind of meaningless, but we walk you through it.

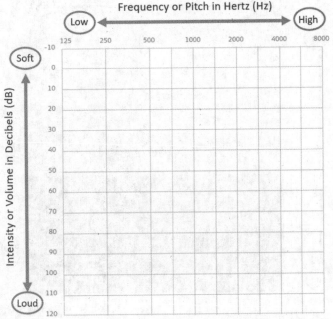

Source: Frank Lin, MD, PhD, and Nicholas Reed, AuD

FIGURE 7-1: A blank audiogram.

Across the top, there are different frequencies or pitches measured in Hertz (Hz) and organized from low- to high-frequency sounds moving left to right. Some people are more familiar with the terms *bass* to represent low-frequency and *treble* to represent high-frequency. An example of a low-frequency sound is thunder roaring during a rainstorm. An example of a high-frequency sound is a tea kettle whistling.

On the left side of the graph are numbers that increase from top to bottom (usually –10 to 120) that represent the intensity or loudness of sound measured in decibels (dB). The greater the number, the louder the sound. Around 0 dB is a sound like leaves rustling in the wind while an ambulance siren is around 120 dB. So, the closer your hearing thresholds are to 0 (or even −10), the better your hearing.

Hearing loss categories on the audiogram

Professionals speak about hearing loss in terms of various categories that describe the degree or severity of hearing loss. Categories are based on your hearing thresholds or how loud sounds need to be for you to hear them. Figure 7-2 shows those categories and the sound intensity ranges in decibels.

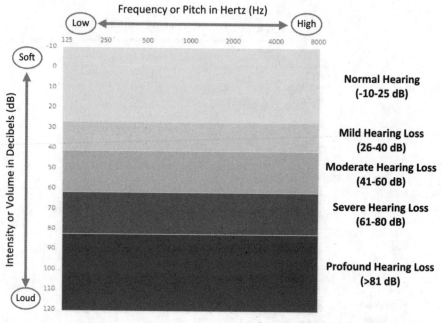

FIGURE 7-2:
The audiogram with categories of hearing loss.

Source: Frank Lin, MD, PhD, and Nicholas Reed, AuD

REMEMBER

Everyone experiences hearing loss differently so it can be difficult to say exactly what each category means for any given person. But broadly speaking, Table 7-1 gives a description of each category and how it relates to speech understanding.

WARNING

Some hearing care providers use terms we don't cover in this book, such as "slight," "moderately severe," or "complete" hearing loss. For this book, we are using the mostly commonly used hearing loss categories used by most clinicians and researchers.

TABLE 7-1:   ## Categories of Hearing Loss

Normal Hearing (Hearing number <25)

Speech should be routinely understandable when spoken clearly

Mild Hearing Loss (Hearing number 25-40)

May experience trouble understanding normal conversation in difficult listening environments like noisy restaurants or when someone's back is turned to you or when someone whispers

Moderate Hearing Loss (Hearing number 41-60)

May have some trouble understanding speech even under the best listening situations

Severe Hearing Loss (Hearing number 61-80)

Speech will be muffled and very difficult to understand, particularly if there are no visual or facial cues

Profound Hearing Loss (Hearing number >80)

Will have a near total inability to understand speech

AM I DEAF? OR IS IT DEAF?

We've all likely used or heard the phrase "Are you deaf?" at some point when we've been exasperated with someone who doesn't appear to be listening. But what in fact does this term mean, and why in some cases is it capitalized?

From a clinical perspective, there actually isn't a precise definition based on a hearing test of when someone is considered to be deaf. More commonly, the term may be applied to people who self-identify as deaf because they can't hear, or have difficulty hearing, spoken language or environmental sounds even when using hearing aids or other hearing technologies. Therefore, two people who have the same objective hearing test results showing a severe hearing loss may have completely different self-assessments of whether they are, in fact, deaf based on their lifestyle and how well they are able to communicate with others.

In contrast, describing yourself as Deaf with a capital "D" means something very different from describing yourself as "deaf." In the former case, Deaf is generally considered to be a linguistic cultural identity generally adopted by individuals born with a severe or profound congenital hearing loss and who communicate via sign language. In the United States, sign language is typically American Sign Language (ASL), but other countries have their own forms of sign language. They may share some similarities with ASL but are completely different (much as Spanish and English are different languages but share some inherent similarities). For people who consider themselves Deaf, deafness is considered part of their identity, and Deaf culture has its own linguistic and social norms. You can find lots more about this in books and information online. You can find lots more about this in books and information online written by members of the Deaf community

Defining Hearing Loss with the Audiogram

After grasping the basic layout of the audiogram, we can put some hearing test results on there and make some sense of them. Figure 7-3 shows an audiogram with the results of a pure-tone hearing test.

The Xs and Os of hearing

On the audiogram (see Figure 7-3), the hearing thresholds are represented by O (right ear) and X (left ear). These are the thresholds obtained with air-conduction testing when the sounds are played through earphones or headphones (in contrast to hearing thresholds obtained with bone conduction testing, which is different and briefly described later).

In Figure 7-3, notice the X and O markings fall into different categories of hearing loss across different frequencies. It is common to have different thresholds at different frequencies. In fact, the vast majority of hearing loss demonstrates a similar pattern, such that with aging, people generally develop poorer hearing in the high frequencies compared to the low frequencies.

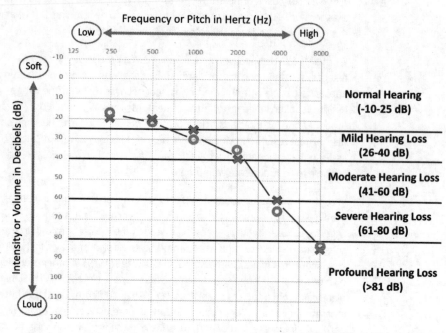

FIGURE 7-3: The audiogram with hearing assessment results.

Source: Frank Lin, MD, PhD, and Nicholas Reed, AuD

CLUTTERED AUDIOGRAMS: OTHER SYMBOLS AND WHAT THEY TELL US ABOUT TYPES OF HEARING LOSS

Your audiogram may resemble a graph of jumbled hieroglyphics. In addition to the Xs and Os from air-conduction testing, you may see symbols such as angle brackets (< >) that represent the bone-conduction results.

You may even see triangles and squares, which represent a technique called *masking* used during your test. In relatively rare cases where someone has large *asymmetries* or differences in hearing between their ears (let's call them a good ear and a bad ear), hearing care professionals will play noise into the good ear while testing the bad ear. This prevents the good ear from compensating for the bad ear (which would give incorrect results).

Interpreting these other symbols is beyond the scope of this book, but suffice it to say that hearing care professionals use these other types of testing methods represented by these symbols to identify the type of hearing loss. There are three types:

- **Sensorineural hearing loss** is the most common type of hearing loss and the focus of this book. It represents the cellular damage in the inner ear. It can be treated with communication strategies (see Chapter 8), hearing aids (see Chapter 9), or even cochlear implants (see Chapter 13), but it is not reversible by any pharmacologic or surgical intervention at this time.

- **Conductive hearing loss** is when sound cannot get to the inner ear to be encoded and sent to the brain. Examples of conductive hearing loss include impacted earwax, fluid in the ears, or a growth in the middle ear space — anything that blocks sound from getting to the inner ear. An otolaryngologist can surgically or medically correct many conductive losses.

- **Mixed hearing loss** is when an individual has both sensorineural and conductive hearing loss. For example, a person may have a mild sensorineural hearing loss but then gets a cold that causes the middle ear space to fill with fluid, which prevents sound from getting to the inner ear. So that person has an added conductive loss on top of their sensorineural hearing loss.

Diving into details of your hearing loss

Professionals use the hearing test results to characterize your hearing loss in terms of degree and pattern of hearing loss.

Degree of hearing loss: Is hearing loss present and, if so, how much?

Your most pressing question following the hearing assessment is likely, "Do I have hearing loss?"

At a most basic level, if a hearing threshold (the Xs and Os), is outside of the normal hearing range (> 25 decibels) on the audiogram, there is some hearing loss present at that specific frequency. Does this mean you have hearing loss if only one frequency has a threshold outside normal? Sort of but not really! Typically, thresholds at multiple frequencies need to be outside of the normal range on the audiogram to be considered significant. But there is no hardline rule for how many.

In Figure 7-3, notice that there are hearing thresholds (Xs and Os) in every category of hearing loss. As we go from low- to high-frequency (left to right), the thresholds get higher in decibel level, which means worse hearing (remember going down on the graph means more hearing loss). Because the thresholds change across frequencies, professionals usually describe the degree of hearing loss by the pattern.

Pattern and range of hearing loss

Going back to Figure 7-3, you can see that the plot has a sloping pattern such that the hearing is normal through the lower-frequencies (250 and 500 Hz) and slopes down to a severe-to-profound loss at the high-frequencies (6,000 and 8,000 Hz). The full description of the audiogram would be *normal sloping to severe/profound hearing loss.* This is audiology jargon for "your hearing loss is fine in low frequencies but is pretty bad in higher frequencies."

REMEMBER

You may find that your hearing care professional comments on how steep the slope of the hearing loss pattern was in test results, using terms such as "gradually sloping" or "precipitously sloping." This refers to how rapid a decline in hearing you have from one frequency to the next. Some people with very steep declines on the audiogram can struggle to adjust to hearing aids, but they can succeed with the right expectations and some extra accessories (see Chapter 12).

Using the audiogram to make sense of how hearing loss affects you

The audiogram is clearly not the easiest way to quickly answer the question of "Do I have hearing loss or not?" But it shines in describing exactly what sounds you are or are not able to hear.

Figure 7-4 is an audiogram of familiar sounds with the same X- and Y-axis labels as Figure 7-1, in that sound goes from low to high frequency going left to right and from soft to loud sound going top to bottom. But this audiogram has pictures representing different sounds. This is like a cheat sheet to help put your hearing loss in perspective relating to what sounds you can and can't hear.

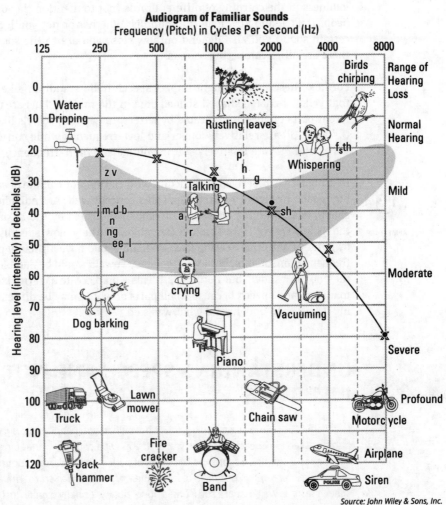

Audiogram of Familiar Sounds
Frequency (Pitch) in Cycles Per Second (Hz)

Source: John Wiley & Sons, Inc.

FIGURE 7-4:
The audiogram of familiar sounds with an overlay of hearing loss results.

Different sounds have different volumes and pitches. For example, in the upper-right corner of Figure 7-4, you see an image of a bird chirping. This sound is **very soft** in volume (indicated by its position near the top of the audiogram) and **high** in pitch (indicated by its position near the right side of the audiogram). Alternatively, in the lower-left corner, you see an image of a lawn mower, which is a **very loud** (near the bottom) and **low-pitched** (near the left side of the audiogram) sound.

In Figure 7-4, we've put the hearing thresholds on the audiogram. In theory, everything on the graph that is above the thresholds is inaudible to the person. So, with this hearing loss, you wouldn't be able to hear rustling leaves, whispering, or birds chirping. But keep in mind that this graph is just a generalization, and whether you can actually hear the sounds depicted on the graph in the real world will vary greatly. For example, there's clear variability in the frequency and loudness in the chirping of different birds (not to mention the loudness at which people talk!), and how loud the sound is. Whether or not you'll be able to hear a certain sound will also depend on how close you are to the sound and whether there are other competing sounds.

For how these results might impact speech understanding, take a closer look at that yellow banana-shaped shaded area in the middle. This area represents different parts of speech, indicated by letters. In general, vowels like "A," "E," "I," O," and "U" are relatively louder and low-frequency while consonants like "F," "SH," and "S" are relatively soft in volume and high-frequency.

REMEMBER

Hearing loss is perceived as difficulty with clarity, not volume of sound. The hearing results in Figure 7-4 represent this concept well. An individual would not be able to hear anything above the thresholds indicated by the Xs and Os. Note that the Xs and Os cut right through the middle of the yellow speech areas (indicated by letters). With this hearing loss, a person would have difficulty perceiving high-frequency consonants, but low-frequency vowels would be audible. So, you'd hear the "no" in "snow" but not the "s." This would create a clarity issue when trying to understand speech because small parts of words may be difficult to hear, making it harder to understand what was said.

UNDERSTANDING SPEECH AND NOT JUST BEEPS

In a diagnostic hearing test, you don't just note when you hear beeps, but you may have also be asked to repeat back some words. If you got a copy of your audiogram, you may see the results of these scores on the sheet of paper. The two most common tests done are the *speech reception threshold* test and the *word recognition score*. There are other speech tests as well that are sometimes done, but we'll briefly explain just these two tests since they're the most commonly done.

The *speech reception threshold* is the softest level at which you can repeat back words. This is reported as a decibel level. A higher number indicates more difficulty repeating words and increased likelihood of hearing loss. The speech reception threshold should match up very closely to the hearing number or pure-tone average (see the later section, "The Hearing Number: An Easier Way to Make Sense of Your Hearing").

The *word recognition score* is the percent of words (generally you'll be read a list of 25 words) repeated back correctly when they are presented at a loud but comfortable listening level. This score ranges from 0 to 100 percent correct. The interpretation of the word recognition score is a little bit tricky and leaves many patients confused. You might get a score of 100 percent and then hear a hearing professional say something like, "Your score of 100 percent makes you a good candidate for hearing aids!"

Wait. What? How can repeating back all the words correctly make you a *good* candidate for hearing aids? It's not intuitive, but remember that the test is done at a louder level, meaning that what it is actually assessing is your ability to hear amplified words. It's not a perfect representation of what hearing aids are like, but the idea is that if you have hearing loss based on the audiogram (see Chapter 6) and do well on the word recognition score, you may be a good candidate for hearing aids.

The Hearing Number: An Easier Way to Make Sense of Your Hearing

The audiogram can be a lot to process. Here we introduce a single number to make your hearing test results much easier to understand and monitor over time. From a clinical perspective, it's called the *pure-tone average,* and more commonly, it's just called the *hearing number.* In a nutshell, the hearing number simply indicates how loud speech sounds have to be for you to hear them. The larger the number, the louder the sounds have to be for you to hear them and hence the poorer your hearing is.

TIP

There's a public health campaign going on now organized by the Johns Hopkins Bloomberg School of Public Health (where both Frank and Nick are based) that's focused on increasing the public's awareness of the importance of knowing their hearing number. Learn more about this campaign and the hearing number at www. hearingnumber.org.

Where the hearing number comes from

You may have noticed that the majority of speech sounds fall between 500 and 4,000 Hz on the audiogram (see Figure 7-4). The hearing number is simply the average of a person's hearing thresholds at these frequencies that span the speech range marked at 500, 1,000, 2,000, and 4,000.

For example, in Figure 7-4, the hearing thresholds for the left ear (Xs on the audiogram) are 20, 25, 40, and 50 dB, respectively, at these four frequencies. The average of these four values is 33.8 (the sum of 20+25+40+50 divided by 4). The pure-tone average, or the hearing number, for the left ear is therefore 33.8.

Doing the same calculation for the right ear (Os on the audiogram) also yields a hearing number, or pure-tone average, that is exactly the same, 33.8. It's really common for both ears to have very similar hearing numbers since both ears typically gradually lose hearing at the same rate with aging.

What the hearing number means to you

Your hearing number in each ear directly indicates how well you can hear speech sounds in that ear and is often used by clinicians and researchers to classify someone's hearing (for example, normal hearing, mild hearing loss, or moderate hearing loss). Figure 7-2 shows commonly used categories of hearing loss that are based on the hearing number and the functional communication challenges that are common with each category of hearing loss.

By monitoring your hearing number periodically (every 1 to 2 years), you can get a clearer sense of how your hearing is changing over time for the sound frequencies that are most important for communication. In many cases, you may not even notice these changes in your hearing because they come on so slowly that it's hard to notice your hearing has changed at all. Knowing your hearing number can provide you with a reality check of whether everyone around you is mumbling a lot more or whether it's in fact your hearing that has changed!

Importantly, in Chapter 4, we discuss the possible effects that hearing loss has on developing poor health outcomes like dementia and falls. If you want to know whether you're possibly at greater risk of developing these conditions, you'll need to know your hearing number!

Previous studies linking hearing loss with these outcomes were all based on the hearing number. In general, these studies have all found that as your hearing number increases, particularly as it gets past 25, you may be at greater risk of developing these outcomes. By keeping track of your hearing number, you'll have a quick objective check of when you may need to consider adopting some of the strategies discussed in this book.

Does my hearing number change?

We mention in Chapter 3 that everyone loses some hearing over time as the inner ear begins to wear out. These changes are directly reflected in changes you'll see in your hearing number over time. Figure 7-5 is an analysis we did at Johns Hopkins of hearing results taken from a large sample of thousands of people of different ages across the United States. When you plot the average hearing number of this group of individuals by age, you can see how the average hearing number worsens over time. Notice that men on average have poorer hearing than women (see Chapter 3).

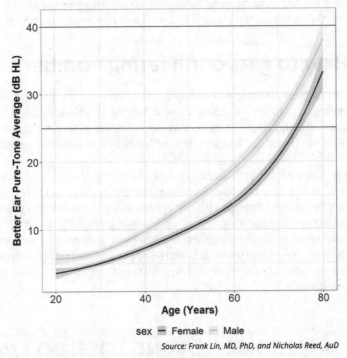

Source: Frank Lin, MD, PhD, and Nicholas Reed, AuD

FIGURE 7-5: Average hearing number by sex for American adults from ages 20–80 years.

Using Figure 7-5 and armed with your hearing number, you can get a sense of whether your hearing number is above or below average for someone of your same age and sex.

What to do with your hearing number

Knowing your own hearing number as well as possibly the hearing number of your spouse or other close family members can cue you in to exactly what you need to do to optimize communication. Later in this book, we discuss the different communication strategies (Chapter 8) and hearing technologies (Chapters 10 and 12) that can be used to optimize your hearing and communication. Knowing which of these strategies and technologies you'll need to consider using can be guided by knowing your hearing number and the general category of hearing loss that your hearing number places you in (refer to Figure 7-2).

More importantly, monitoring your hearing number over time can give you the best sense of how well you're able to hear and engage with the world around you. You may already have a sense of some of your other key health metrics — for example, your blood pressure or, if you have diabetes, your blood sugar level. Each of these metrics gives you an indication of your health and what you may need to do. Knowing your hearing number similarly empowers you to better understand your hearing and the steps you can take to optimize your hearing.

How to get your hearing number

You or your hearing professional can calculate your hearing number from the audiogram simply by adding up your hearing thresholds at 500, 1,000, 2,000, and 4,000 Hz and dividing by 4. You can calculate a hearing number for both your right ear (indicated by Os on the audiogram) and your left ear (Xs).

TIP

You can also get your hearing number directly from many smartphone apps as well. At the time this book went to press, the Apple iPhone platform offers an easy way to do this through either the native Apple Health app (choose the Hearing option and then audiogram) or with apps such as Mimi and SonicCloud through your Apple or Android app store. More apps are expected to become available in the next one to two years on both the Apple and Android platforms that will allow you to take a pure-tone hearing test and get your hearing number on your smartphone.

I HAVE SOME HEARING LOSS. DO I *NEED* HEARING AIDS?

In all aspects of healthcare, including hearing health, we use categories with different cut points to define conditions. These cut points are defined based on population-level data, which doesn't always apply neatly across the board to the individual level. In the case of hearing loss and hearing aids, this means that generally everyone with a hearing number above 25 could benefit from hearing aids. But at the individual level, whether you would benefit enough from hearing aids and whether you truly **need** them is determined on a case-by-case basis.

No two people react to hearing loss the same way. Remember that hearing involves both the ear and the brain. One person with a mild hearing loss may not notice it affect their life at all as they are able to completely compensate, while another person with that same hearing loss may need a handheld amplifier in particularly tough listening situations, while a third person with the same hearing loss simply cannot get by without hearing aids.

Many people see hearing care as a limited option of getting hearing aids or nothing, but the reality is hearing care spans a continuum of ways to address hearing loss depending on your specific needs. This includes:

- Avoiding difficult listening situations
- Applying simple communication strategies
- Asking for what you need at home, at work, and in social situations
- Using a personal sound amplifier for one or two specific situations
- OTC hearing aids for mild and moderate losses
- Trying prescription hearing aids for more severe losses
- Using accessories for hearing aids to help get through the most difficult listening situations
- Using a smartphone speech-to-text app
- Getting cochlear implants

So, no, you don't *need* necessarily hearing aids just because you have hearing loss, but we encourage you to consider all your hearing care options. These options are all discussed later in this book.

WARNING

If you're obtaining your hearing number on your own through the various hearing testing apps that are available on smartphones, be warned that not all tests are the same. There are lots of different ways of doing a hearing test, and some apps might give you some sort of "hearing score" or hearing percentage. It's hard to say that these numbers mean. You'll want to stick with an app that clearly tells you that the number it is giving you is based on an average of your hearing thresholds at 500, 1,000, 2,000, and 4,000 Hz.

TIP

For the most up-to-date information about smartphone apps with which you can test and obtain your own hearing number at home, check out www.hearingnumber.org.

Guiding Your Hearing Health Journey with Your Results

Whether you've looked at your test results through the lens of the audiogram or the hearing number, you've learned something about your hearing and now have an idea of where you stand. But what do you actually do with this information? The following sections explain.

Monitor changes in hearing

Everyone's hearing gets worse over time, but often you may not realize it because it comes on so slowly. When you understand your hearing test results, and more importantly your hearing number, you can self-monitor your own hearing and have a clearer idea of when you need to take action based on these results as well as what you're experiencing on a daily basis.

Without knowing and monitoring your hearing number over time, it's easy to just shrug off any hearing problems you may be having and attribute the problem to others not speaking clearly. As we talk about in Chapter 2, though, the experience of feeling like others are mumbling and not speaking clearly is exactly what hearing loss leads to.

TIP

Make sure you store or record your hearing test results somewhere safe. It's important to always have a baseline hearing test with follow-up tests so that you can keep an eye on how your hearing is changing over time.

Use it or lose it

After a patient has been tested and asks about seeking treatment, some hearing care professionals will respond with the phrase, "Use it or lose it." What they mean is that delaying or not treating hearing loss now may make it more difficult to optimize your hearing and ability to communicate later.

When we have hearing loss, the ear may send garbled sounds that are difficult to process, or the brain may stop receiving some sounds altogether. When the brain doesn't receive sound from the ear for long periods or you get accustomed to no longer trying to listen, the brain may gradually lose the ability to process these sounds efficiently.

Think of your brain like a muscle; if you don't use a muscle, it will atrophy over time, and when you need it again, it will be tough to use and may not be as strong. This is what professionals mean when they urge you to address hearing loss sooner rather than later. Knowing the results of your hearing test and hearing number can cue you in to when it's time to act. We go over all the different communication strategies and hearing technologies you can use to address hearing loss in the later parts of this book.

3

Taking Charge of Your Hearing

Discover everyday straregies to overcome hearing loss.

Recognize how a hearing aid works.

Review your hearing aid options and how to navigate the hearing aid marketplace.

Appreciate creating routines and strategies to optimize hearing aid use.

Introduce technology that can improve how hearing aids work for you.

Understand medical and surgical options for specific types of hearing loss.

Chapter 8

Fine-Tuning Your Life to Hearing Loss

D o you recall ever having to deal with a finnicky radio dial on an analog clock-radio when trying to tune in a specific radio station? Or perhaps, you may be more familiar with having to adjust the tuning pegs on a guitar to make sure the G string is actually a "G" and not verging toward a "G sharp." If so, you're familiar with the exact idea of adjusting or fine-tuning something until it sounds just right.

We love this metaphor for hearing and communication because the same principle applies! Everyone — and that means you, your family members, and your friends — will gradually lose some hearing over time. The radio will come in a little fuzzy; that G string will sound a little off. How can we get it right? We all need to hear well to communicate with others and engage with everything else we do in life.

In this chapter, we focus on communication strategies that you can use on a daily basis to help manage hearing loss as well as everyday technologies that you likely have access to or may already use. We also review resources for advocating for yourself and seeking out support groups and networks if you need them.

Discovering Where Adjustments Can Be Made

Everyday strategies to improve hearing focus on either improving the quality of sounds that get to the ear or providing additional cues to the brain to help it "decode" the signal that comes from the ear:

>> **Sound quality:** For example, a clear voice in a quiet room is *very* different from a voice coming to you from across a large table at a busy, crowded restaurant. Communication and technological strategies can increase sound quality to improve hearing.

>> **Brain decoding:** The brain decodes the auditory signal into meaning. The brain not only uses the auditory signals from the ears but also relies on other visual cues (such as lip movements) and contextual cues (such as other words in the sentence). Communication and technological strategies can provide the brain with additional information to aid the brain in interpreting the incoming sounds.

Read on to find strategies that can help you in different hearing situations and allow you to make positive changes for yourself.

Finding No-Tech Communication Strategies for Everyday Situations

Communication strategies focus on improving the quality of the sound you hear or helping your brain get the additional visual or contextual information that can help it decode sound that enters the ears. The following sections contain strategies that you can employ right away to help you hear better.

Get close

Being closer to the person you want to hear is always better.

How close, you say? Being at arm's length for a conversation is ideal.

Sound loudness and quality both drop off quickly with increasing distance from the speaker. In particular, in certain rooms with high ceilings or lots of hard surfaces, there can be a lot of echo or reverberation, which can rapidly degrade the quality of the voice you actually want to hear if you're farther from the speaker.

While it's not always possible to be at arm's length (such as when listening to a speaker in a lecture room or attending religious services), you'll still want to be as close as you can to the person you're trying to hear. Sitting in the front row rather than the back of the room in these settings can make all the difference between understanding everything that is said versus only catching every few words.

Likewise, don't try talking to someone when they're in a different room of the house. Being in the same room will make communication far easier.

Be face-to-face

Being at arm's length would seem to imply also being face-to-face, and while this may often be the case, it's not always true. For example, imagine speaking with someone sitting next to you at a dinner table versus someone sitting directly across from you at the same table. While both speakers may be close to you, you may find that it's easier to understand the person sitting across from you.

The reason for this is that being face-to-face with the speaker allows your brain to also access the visual cues of lip movements and facial expressions as your brain is working to decode in real-time the incoming sounds. These cues are hugely helpful for allowing your brain to quickly interpret sounds into meaning.

You may not realize it, but you have been learning a form of lip-reading since childhood (see Chapter 2). Babies learn to make certain sounds by seeing lip and mouth movements, and toddlers learn language by naturally watching people's faces. Humans are exquisitely tuned to reading facial expressions conveying emotions, and these facial expressions are virtually universal across all human societies despite the vast cultural differences that may separate two random people on Earth. These emotional visual cues help your brain understand what you are hearing. By facing the person you're speaking with and taking in visual cues, you give yourself an advantage to hearing and understanding what is being said to you.

Summarize and repeat ("Huhs" don't help!)

You may have noticed that both you and nearly every other person have a tendency to immediately reply with a "Huh?" or "What?" after not understanding something that was spoken.

The person on the receiving end of the "Huh?" will then generally repeat back what was said, hopefully with more success. For individuals with hearing loss, this reflexive "Huh?" can seem like a constant process throughout the day. And for those on the receiving end of the "Huh?" — which may be an increasingly frustrated spouse or family member — the "Huhs?" over time can exacerbate the situation.

There has to be a better option, right?

YES!

TIP

Next time, you're in this situation, rather than saying "Huh?" or "What?" it's far more helpful to quickly summarize what you did hear and ask for clarification.

For example, if your spouse is asking you on the phone to pick up a few items while you're at the grocery store but you only caught a few words around "milk" and "bread," you could say, "I heard you say milk and bread, but I missed the rest."

This makes it a lot easier for the speaker, who now knows exactly what to repeat. Importantly, it also shows the speaker that you were actually trying to listen (rather than purposely ignoring the speaker, as many spouses complain!).

Optimizing Your Listening Environment

To improve sound quality and the cues that your brain uses to understand sound, there are also strategies that you should know about to optimize the environment for listening.

Turn down any background sounds

Turning down background noise may be obvious, but it's often forgotten about. The sound quality of whatever you're trying to hear — whether it's a friend's voice or the dialog from a movie — will be much better if there aren't other sounds competing with it. These other sounds can directly interfere with the voice you want to hear or make it much harder for your brain to distinguish the voice you're trying to hear.

In your home, this means routinely turning down any sound sources to try to isolate what you're trying to hear. For example, when trying to talk to someone in your home, this could include routinely doing the following:

>> Muting, turning down, or turning off the TV or music

>> Closing the laundry room door if the washer or dryer is running

>> Turning off the faucet if you're trying to hear someone while doing dishes

>> Moving to a different area of the home that is quieter if you can't directly turn down background sounds

The hard part about these strategies is remembering to do them on a regular basis and reminding your communication partner to do the same.

Avoid reverberation

Reverberation means the natural echoing of sounds as they bounce off walls and other surfaces — the longer the reverberation time, the longer you'll hear the sound even after the sound source stops. If you've ever been in an old cavernous cathedral with an organ, you may be able to imagine this sense of reverberation.

Sometimes reverberation is a good thing. For example, if you're in a concert hall listening to music, acoustical engineers design the concert hall in a certain way to have a precise degree of reverberation. This gives music the richness and fullness that you're used to hearing with music.

In contrast, reverberation is terrible when it comes to understanding speech. These echoes degrade the quality of speech sounds tremendously, making it much harder for your brain to decode the sound.

REMEMBER

A lot of factors go into whether a room has more or less reverberation, but the key things to keep in mind are

>> Lower ceilings and smaller rooms help *reduce* reverberation.

>> Soft surfaces (such as rugs, drapes, pillows, upholstered furniture, and carpeted floors) all *reduce* reverberation.

These suggestions are important to keep in mind because they can affect not only how you choose to arrange your own home but also how you pick out a restaurant or which room you want to be in while at a party.

Pick the right restaurants

Oy vey . . . restaurants are tough and perhaps the bane of any person with a hearing loss. A lot of characteristics are common to restaurants that make hearing and communication hard:

- » Dining rooms with high ceilings and lots of hard surfaces, such as tile floors and metal tables.

- » Lots of people are talking at once.

- » Background music. Restaurant managers know a certain "din" in the dining room (and particularly in bars) can help create a desired livelier atmosphere and encourage faster turnover of tables.

- » Low levels of lighting. Dim lights can lend a more intimate atmosphere but can hinder your ability to see other people's faces clearly (and read the menu!).

All these factors conspire to muddy sound quality and affect the visual cues that enable your brain to "hear" better.

If you've been dealing with a hearing loss for years and have had to navigate dynamic social situations at restaurants, just reading this list may be making your heart beat faster and your palms a bit sweaty. These situations can be stressful! And precisely the exact opposite of what a night out for dinner should be about.

TIP

Fortunately, with some careful planning, these challenges can be overcome. Here are the key tips to keep in mind:

- » When possible, pick a restaurant with lower ceilings and lots of soft surfaces (for example, rugs, carpets, drapes, and soft upholstered furniture).

- » Choose a time of day when the dining room is less busy.

- » Call ahead and request a table in an area that is quieter, has better lighting, and is ideally in a corner or against a wall. The restaurant host may not always pick the right area, but increasingly, we find that restaurants are getting this request often enough that they have a sense of what works.

- » Sit with your back to the wall or in the corner when possible. This reduces the amount of noise coming at you from behind.

- » Sit across from the person you most need to hear. Being directly across from the speaker allows you to get the full benefit of facial cues and is where the sound quality is the best.

- » In a group, sit directly next to the person you're most accustomed to listening to. This may often be a spouse or other close family member or friend. The position of this speaker, where you won't have immediate access to visual cues and where the voice is primarily coming to only one ear, is the hardest for you to understand. Your brain will be more accustomed to decoding this person's voice, and this individual will also hopefully be most familiar with how to best communicate with you (if someone needs some communication coaching, check out Chapter 14!).

NOISY RESTAURANTS: A PURPOSEFUL PROBLEM WITH EMERGING TECH SOLUTIONS

Restaurants are loud and notoriously difficult listening environments. Not only does this make conversation tough, but it presents a safety issue. Noise levels in some restaurants at peak hours are dangerously loud and could damage hearing with enough exposure. Part of the noise problem is to be expected due to poor acoustic design and just the fact that the presence of a lot of people talking is, well, noisy. But, to some extent, the loud noise is by design as restauranteurs want to present a hip and lively atmosphere, but it has clearly gotten out of control.

Some of the noise can be addressed by turning down the background music or adding sound dampening materials to reduce noise. One cutting edge company, Meyer Sound (www.meyersound.com), has introduced a combination of high-quality acoustic design with electronic sound engineering solutions to reduce noise and allow for clear, intimate conversations at your table while maintaining the lively restaurant ambiance regardless of how jam-packed or sparsely occupied the restaurant is. The result is a balanced high-quality sound experience where you can get the best of both worlds.

While we wait for the new tech to catch on, you can also take action and seek out quieter restaurants. But how? SoundPrint (www.soundprint.com) has been called "the Yelp of noise ratings." This smartphone app allows people to rate noise levels in various locations, including restaurants, and even take actual noise level ratings with their phone! With this app you can look at noise ratings for restaurants across your community and seek out quieter locations for a better dining experience.

Using Everyday Technology Strategies

When people think of technology strategies for hearing, hearing aids and other specialized technologies like cochlear implants may come to mind. These technologies are great and are covered in greater detail in other chapters in Part 3, but importantly, there are a multitude of everyday technologies that you may already have access to that can be used to optimize hearing and communication.

Closed captioning

We love closed captions! Both of the authors are still young enough to not yet appreciably have any noticeable hearing problems, but we still rely on these all the time when watching TV or movies.

Captions (also known as subtitles) on TV are mandated by federal policy in the United States and many other countries. Captions are generally available with both live TV (for example, news shows and sporting events) and prerecorded movies and shows. This feature is built into nearly all televisions and is also available on digital streaming services such as Amazon, Apple TV, Disney Plus, HBO Max, Hulu, and Netflix. You can generally find a button on your TV remote labeled "CC" or a menu option for "CC," subtitles, or closed captioning to activate this feature.

In general, you'll find that captioning for prerecorded shows or movies are superb and mesh exactly with the spoken words. In contrast, captioning for live TV will be slightly delayed and with imperfect accuracy because these captions are actually appearing "live" in contrast to prerecorded content where there is more time to ensure accuracy. Much of this live transcription is now being done by automated speech recognition systems, which are getting better and better but still make mistakes at times.

Closed captions are great mainly because they make it so much easier to understand what is being said and allow your brain to not have to concentrate as hard to catch the dialog. For some people, seeing the captions on the screen takes a bit of getting used to at first, but if you're like most people, they rapidly become indispensable.

Captions come into play not only with TV shows and movies but also increasingly with video calls, specialized captioned phones, and smartphone apps that can be used during in-person conversations. You can find out more about captioning in these unique settings in Chapter 12.

Voice over internet protocol (VOIP) calls and videocalls

Traditional phone calls made over a landline or a cellular phone are good, but you may have noticed that the quality of the speaker's voice often isn't that great.

For example, when his kids were young, Frank routinely couldn't tell apart the voice of his son or daughter because they sounded so similar over the phone (but completely different in person!).

The source of this confusion has to do with the fact that most landline or cellphone calls have a frequency range for sound transmission that's limited to 300 Hz to about 3,000 Hz. The majority of speech sounds occur all the way up to 6,000–8,000 Hz, which means some parts of speech are lost on these regular phone calls.

In other words, a regular phone call is working against you from the get-go by lowering the quality of the voices you want to hear. Much of this is because of the limitations of the relatively dated technology used for landline and cell-phone calls.

Fortunately, there's a solution!

Phone calls made over VOIP (voice over internet protocol) services such as FaceTime, Google Voice, Skype, WhatsApp, and Zoom all typically have wideband audio. This means that the frequency range of sounds being transmitted on the phone call can extend from 50 to 7,000 Hz, which makes the sound quality *so* much better. You'll notice when making a call on any of these services that voices sound more full or lifelike. This improved sound quality can make a huge difference with speech understanding, particularly if you have some hearing loss that has developed over time.

Getting started with using VOIP services couldn't be easier. Just download the preferred app on your smartphone or computer and follow the instructions to get started. Many of these services are completely free but do require you to have an internet connection on your smartphone or computer.

You may have even spoken to someone over one of these VOIP services and not realized it. If you've ever spoken to someone over a computer, a smart speaker such as Amazon Alexa or Google Home, or a smartphone where you used FaceTime, Google Voice, Skype, WhatsApp, or Zoom, you've been on a VOIP call!

An added benefit of many of the computer or phone apps that allow for VOIP is that they may also allow for video calls as well (such as FaceTime, Skype, What'sApp, and Zoom). Having both the video component (with visual and lip cues) and the audio signal can make it a lot easier for you to understand speech.

Speaking Up for Yourself

Hearing loss has often been described as an "invisible" disability. Other sensory or physical impairments, such as blindness or a mobility impairment requiring a wheelchair, are often immediately obvious to others. But having a subtle degree of hearing loss is often not apparent to others, and hence, they may not understand how to accommodate your communication needs.

While thinking of hearing loss as being an invisible disability may resonate with some readers, other people with hearing loss may be taken aback as being identified as someone with a "disability" or having particular communication needs.

For them, hearing loss has nothing to do with their identity, and they certainly don't need to be treated any differently.

Where you fall on this spectrum may influence to some degree what it means to advocate for yourself and how you feel comfortable doing it.

Regardless of where you are on this spectrum, the key factor to keep in mind with any form of self-advocacy is that you just want to be able to communicate effectively with others.

In situations where you're having trouble understanding someone because you can't hear them well, there are two things you can do:

1. Let the other person know you may be having trouble hearing them.

2. Suggest a solution.

Ways to identify that you're having trouble hearing

Letting the other person know you're having trouble hearing may sound intimidating, but there are a bunch of different ways to do this depending on what you're comfortable with. If you don't feel comfortable explicitly identifying yourself as having a hearing loss, use these more neutral ways of expressing this same idea:

>> "I can't hear you well because of all the noise in this room."

>> "I missed what you said because of the other people talking."

>> "That music is so loud I didn't catch what you said."

Giving the speaker a solution

The next step you can take is to offer the speaker a pragmatic solution. To do this, you have to know exactly what strategies will in fact help you communicate better. In the vast majority of cases, the other person won't know what to do unless you tell them. What you say depends on the situation. Examples of these include the following:

>> **At a noisy cocktail party:** "I can't hear you well because of the noise in this room. Let's step into the hallway to talk."

>> **Over dinner at a restaurant:** "I missed what you said because of all the racket in this restaurant. Could you please speak more slowly?"

>> **At a doctor's appointment:** "I have trouble hearing you when you're facing the computer. Would you be able to face me when you speak?"

The keys with this situational self-advocacy strategy are telling the person there's a problem and offering a proactive solution.

Practicing self-advocacy

Self-advocacy is complex and requires that you know the state of your hearing, what you need to function at home and in the world, and even your rights as someone with hearing loss (which we address in Chapter 16). Hopefully this book helps you build that foundational knowledge or get started on that path.

We all react differently to different situations and many of the situations where you will most need to self-advocate will be stressful. An example might be when you're communicating with a doctor in a hospital — an already stressful situation that can be exacerbated if you have trouble hearing. Self-advocacy comes easier with a commitment to yourself to ask for what you need and practice. Here are some suggestions:

>> Anticipate your needs in a situation and make a plan ahead of time.

>> Try not to rely on someone else to advocate for you. Many people may think they are helping when they are advocating for you. Be aware of when others take on that role and let them know that you are happy for their support but that you will be advocating for yourself.

>> Practice explaining your needs to a trusted companion or in low-risk settings with friends and family.

>> Experiment with what approach, words, and tone work for you.

>> Find a role model and support group. It can be helpful to learn from others with hearing loss how they have advocate for themselves.

REMEMBER

Self-advocacy is extremely important. Not everyone fully understands your hearing like you do, and no one understands your needs better than you do. Taking the time to explain those needs helps you while spreading awareness of hearing loss. In fact, by educating one individual on your needs today, you might improve an experience for someone with hearing loss tomorrow.

Reading about others with hearing loss

There's a lot more to self-advocacy that goes well beyond the scope of this book. Needless to say, a lot of people have struggled in private for years, feeling embarrassment, shame, and frustration at not being able to communicate well with others because of a hearing loss. The strategies in this chapter and the rest of this book are given with the hope that this information will equip you to avoid this fate. By reading this book, you are standing up for your right to a better quality of life.

We also recommend a couple of other great books written by people we've known who have had hearing loss as an adult. Their books go over their journeys with hearing loss, including all the challenges they have faced and the strategies that have worked for them. If you're worried that hearing loss is increasingly defining who you are and what you can and cannot do, reading about these authors' first-person accounts on what they have experienced may be eye-opening and helpful. They are

>> *Hear & Beyond: Live Skillfully with Hearing Loss* by Shari Eberts and Gael Hannan (published by Page Two)

>> *Shouting Won't Help* by Katherine Bouton (published by Picador Paper)

Seeking Out Support Groups

Not everyone with hearing loss needs a support group. That being said, as with anything in life, being with like-minded peers who have faced similar experiences and challenges can be helpful.

If you're finding that hearing loss is increasingly something you're worried about for yourself or others, finding a support group to discuss these concerns may help. There are many different types of advocacy organizations focused on hearing loss, and they differ in terms of their constituency — that is, the type of hearing loss that their members have.

The most relevant one for the readers of this book is likely the Hearing Loss Association of America (HLAA; www.hearingloss.org), whose members are primarily those who have developed hearing loss as adults. The main priorities of HLAA members are simply to be able to communicate optimally with others and to engage with the world. The HLAA does some great work and has regional chapters around the country where members periodically get together to discuss concerns and share strategies for communicating well.

Other organizations focus on other types of hearing loss. For example, the National Association of the Deaf (NAD; www.nad.org) advocates for individuals who are culturally Deaf and primarily use sign language to communicate. Other organizations such as the Alexander Graham Bell Association for the Deaf and Hard of Hearing (www.agbell.org) primarily focus on pediatric hearing loss.

TIP

No local HLAA chapter or other formal support group near you? Identify a friend or family member who can be your go-to hearing-support partner. Or ask your local hearing care professional to put you in contact with others with hearing loss who might want to form an informal support group. It can be helpful to have someone to talk to about hearing loss — even if just to bounce ideas for addressing difficult listening situations off one another and receive some reassurance from shared lived experiences.

Chapter **9**

Looking at How Hearing Aids Work

We bet that if you're reading this book, one of your primary interests is learning more about hearing aids. It makes sense — many of us immediately think about hearing aids when we think about hearing loss. But here's the thing: Most of us know next to nothing about what hearing aids actually do.

In this chapter, we take a dive into how hearing aids work and what they look like (hint: they've come a long way since their inception). And we give you the good and the not-so-good points of the different styles.

Understanding Hearing Aids

Today's hearing aids are amazing pieces of technology that magnify and manipulate sound for a custom output to meet the wearer's hearing needs. But it hasn't always been this way.

Humankind has been working on devices to help overcome hearing loss for centuries — all the way back to the ear trumpet in the 17th century. Electric-powered hearing aids were introduced in the early 20th century but were not portable devices. By the mid-20th century, the invention of transistors allowed for smaller devices that could be worn on-person. We've seen an explosion of technology since then. Some modern hearing aids pack the same computing power as a laptop in a sleek device tiny enough to completely hide behind your ear!

The anatomy of a hearing aid: How hearing aids work

Hearing aids are designed to make sound louder and clearer based on the wearer's hearing needs. At a basic level, all hearing aids have three main parts in the process of amplifying sound (see Figure 9-1):

>> First, a microphone on the outside of the hearing aid picks up the sound in your environment.

>> Second, an amplifier built into the body of the hearing aid makes that sound louder.

>> Third, a receiver or speaker sends the signal into your ear.

Most modern hearing aids have a fourth part: a processor that analyzes the sounds in the environment. The processor can be thought of as the brains of the hearing aid. It works with the amplifier to manipulate the sound in very specific ways to customize the sound for its owner's hearing loss.

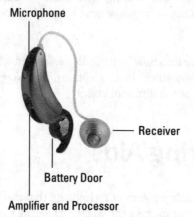

Microphone

Receiver

Battery Door

FIGURE 9-1:
The basic parts of a hearing aid.

Amplifier and Processor

Source: John Wiley & Sons, Inc.

Hearing aids don't make all sounds louder

A common misconception is that hearing aids simply make everything louder. But hearing loss is not so simple that increasing volume automatically improves audibility. In fact, increasing all sound can make it even more difficult for someone with hearing loss to understand speech and other environmental sounds. The hearing aid's job is to amplify sounds that a person has a difficult time hearing. This is an oversimplification, but we like to think of it like this: If you were at dinner with a very soft-spoken person and a loud talker, the hearing aid would add a lot of volume to the soft-spoken person's voice while leaving the loud talker's voice alone or adding minimal volume to it.

Each person's hearing pattern is unique. We all have a hearing perception range from the softest sound we can recognize to the point where sound becomes too loud for us to tolerate. Scientifically, this is known as your *dynamic range of sound.*

An interesting phenomenon with hearing loss is that it affects your ability to perceive sounds that are too soft for your own hearing levels while at the other end of that range, the loudness tolerance remains the same. So, what was loud before you developed hearing loss is still loud. This means that hearing loss causes the range from what is too soft to what is too loud to shrink. Professionals call this *reduced dynamic range.* Hearing aids adjust to your reduced dynamic range by making certain soft sounds louder, while leaving already loud sounds alone.

Let's put that all together with an example. Imagine you're in your house during a summer rainstorm. There's a full range of sounds: the soft sound of the wind whooshing by your window, a medium sound of the steady thump of raindrops hitting your house, and the loud crashes of thunder. Someone with a reduced dynamic range from hearing loss can't hear the wind at all, can just barely hear the raindrops, but can hear the thunder as loud as before. What was once a medium sound for people with normal hearing is now a soft sound for those with hearing loss but loud is still loud — it's a smaller range. This illustrates how sounds can rapidly go from soft to too loud for individuals with hearing loss — a startling experience. In this case, hearing aids would add a lot of volume to the wind, just a little volume to the raindrops, but leave the thunder alone. See Figure 9-2.

TECHNICAL STUFF

You can imagine that it is very difficult to find the balance to make sounds loud but not too loud. *Compression* is the technical term for the modern process that hearing aids use to make soft sounds louder while not changing the already loud sounds in order to stay within an individual's dynamic range.

REMEMBER

Hearing aids don't just focus on what's soft and loud; they also consider different frequencies or pitches of sound. Hearing loss doesn't occur equally across different frequencies. The vast majority of hearing loss affects the ability to hear higher frequencies like a whistle while the ability to hear low frequencies like a bass drum remains relatively normal or near normal. Therefore, hearing aids are customized to each individual's hearing pattern and apply volume only at the specific frequencies needed for that individual.

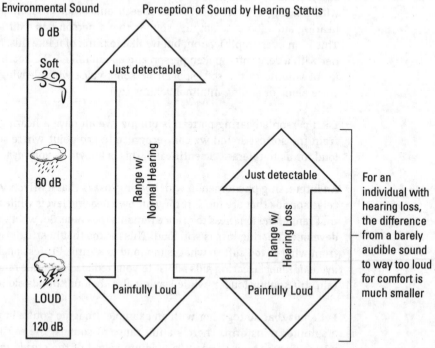

Environmental Sound   Perception of Sound by Hearing Status

FIGURE 9-2:
Dynamic range.

Source: John Wiley & Sons, Inc.

Enhancing clarity of sound with hearing aids

Most hearing loss is due to the deterioration of cells in the ear (see Chapter 3). Currently, there is no way to restore these cells. This means that hearing aids are still delivering sound to damaged cells. So while making sound louder, many hearing aids also boost clarity. They do this by augmenting what you want to hear while dampening sounds you don't want to hear.

TECHNICAL STUFF

The name of the game in enhancing clarity focuses on what is referred to as the *signal to noise ratio*. This is the ratio of the sound you want to hear (the signal) to what you don't want to hear (noise).

Sound is personal

We all have our own preferences for sounds, and every situation is unique. One person's noise is another person's music. For example, at the time of writing this sentence, coauthor Nick's toddler is sitting next to him. If Nick's toddler were to cry, most other people could ignore the noise as it doesn't have a specific meaning to them. But for Nick, his toddler's cries are an important sound that indicates he needs to give the child immediate attention. Even if he doesn't like the sound of crying, he needs to hear it loud and clear. So, do hearing aids really know what you want to hear? The short answer is no. The longer answer is that hearing aids are technologically advanced pieces of equipment that have become really good at identifying what you likely want to hear, while stopping short of being able to think for you.

How hearing aids pick out sounds

In this section, we dig into the features a hearing aid uses to distinguish important sounds versus unimportant noise.

The first way many hearing aids decide what is an interesting sound worth focusing on is by analyzing where that sound comes from. Many hearing aids have a feature called *directionality*. With this feature, the hearing aid amplifies sounds in front of the wearer while dampening sounds behind the wearer. The concept is rooted in the idea that people usually turn their heads and look at the sounds they want to hear. Directionality is particularly useful in settings with multiple talkers, such as restaurants.

But the setting isn't permanent because sometimes we want to hear sounds regardless of where they come from. The directionality mode can be switched on and off. In fact, many modern hearing aids have the option to automatically switch back and forth from the directionality mode to an *omnidirectional* mode, which amplifies all sounds equally regardless of location relative to the hearing aid user. This depends on how much noise is in the environment. For example, your hearing aids would switch to directionality mode in a noisy restaurant while remaining in omnidirectional mode when bird-watching in a quiet forest.

The second way hearing aids try to distinguish what is an interesting sound worth focusing on is by identifying speech using *advanced signal processing techniques.* Speech is dynamic. When people speak, their voices rise or soften to put emphasis on different words. There are pauses of different lengths between words and sentences. Speech speeds up rapidly if the speaker is excited and slows down when the speaker wants to make a point. Hearing aids can identify these unique patterns and focus on amplifying speech above all other sounds. Conversely, if a sound is not dynamic but rather steady, like the hum of an electric appliance, the hearing aid may ignore that sound completely.

TIP

Although a hearing aid can distinguish signals of interest, keep in mind that it might not always tune into what you, personally, want to hear. A good mindset to have during your hearing aid journey is to remember that the hearing aid is not infallible and will require refinement to be customized to your preferences. You may still have difficulty hearing in a specific situation even with your hearing aids. Rather than avoiding that situation in the future, try talking to a professional about the situation and your experience because there are ways to reprogram the hearing aid for success the next time. Check out Chapter 10 for information on how to pick out a hearing aid.

WARNING

Hearing aids are very useful, but not quite perfect. Remember, they're just machines designed to help you as best they can. How the hearing aid amplifies and manipulates sound is different from how your brain processes that sound. Ultimately, hearing aids cannot restore hearing to "normal" and it takes time to adjust to the sound. We talk about realistic expectations and good habits to maximize the benefits from hearing aids in Chapter 11.

Checking Out the Different Styles of Hearing Aids

Modern hearing aids are sleek, and many styles are nearly invisible. This is a far cry from early hearing aids that required body-worn accessories (to visualize that, imagine something like the old Discman CD player worn on your belt with wires attached to headphones). It's also a far cry from the mental image many people have when they picture hearing aids as large and bulky pieces of plastic that stick out from behind the ear connected to huge earpieces sitting in your ear canal.

REMEMBER

Hearing aids come in several different shapes and sizes to customize the fit to the wearer. For the purposes of this book, we cover the broad-style categories but always remember that other variants exist and different manufacturers use different names. Generally, there are two main styles of hearing aids: behind-the-ear and in-the-ear. Each has some subtypes.

TIP

A good hearing aid fit is important to prevent that buzzing sound that is known as feedback. This happens when the amplified sound coming out of the hearing aid speaker is picked up again by the hearing aid microphone and reamplified.

Behind-the-ear

Behind-the-ear hearing aids, often known as BTEs, are the most common style of hearing aid. The hearing aid sits behind the ear — hence, the name — while a tube runs to the front of the ear where it connects to either an earmold or dome in the wearer's ear canal, as shown in Figure 9-3. While earmolds are custom made to fit a wearer's ear, domes are premade mushroom-shaped silicone pieces that come variety of sizes and designs to find the best fit for the wearer's ear canal. BTEs have evolved into several subtypes, each with its own advantages and disadvantages.

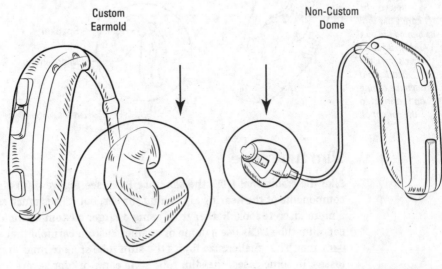

Custom Earmold

Non-Custom Dome

Source: John Wiley & Sons, Inc.

FIGURE 9-3: Earmolds versus domes.

WARNING

Earmolds require a custom impression of your ear canal. There are at-home, do-it-yourself earmold impression kits, but we recommend you use these with caution. Improper use can leave silicone material in the ear which requires a professional to remove. When in doubt, see a hearing care professional to make your earmold impressions.

Traditional BTEs

The *traditional* BTE (see Figure 9-4) houses all the components of the hearing aid (the microphone, amplifier, processor, and speaker) in a single space that sits behind the ear. It is connected to a custom earmold using flexible, medical-grade plastic tubing. The BTE is a fairly rugged product that provides ample space for more powerful hardware, which can accommodate the needs of any degree of hearing loss. There are even "power" models for profound hearing loss.

While the traditional BTE is the most versatile of hearing aid design, it has not always been perceived as the most discrete, so engineers have come up with newer versions of the BTE: slim tube and receiver-in-the-canal BTEs.

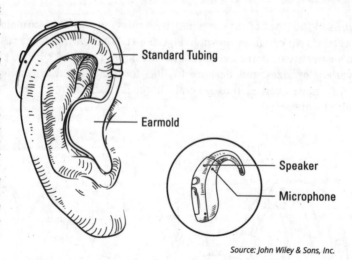

FIGURE 9-4:
Traditional
behind the ear
(BTE) hearing aid.
Note: *All
components
(microphone,
speaker, amplifier,
and processer) are
encased within the
body of the
hearing aid that
sits behind the ear.
Amplified sound
travels from the
hearing aid
through the tubing
and earmold to
the ear canal.*

Standard Tubing

Earmold

Speaker

Microphone

Source: John Wiley & Sons, Inc.

Slim tube style

Like the traditional BTE, the *slim tube* BTE (see Figure 9-5) also houses all the components of the hearing aid behind the ear, but it uses much smaller tubing for a more discrete look. Rather than using a larger custom earmold that fills up the ear, slim tube BTEs use a dome or smaller custom earmold that sits deeper in the ear canal. The smaller size limits the slim tube style to mild to moderate hearing losses. In some cases, the slim tube style can work for severe hearing loss, but it is pushing the boundaries of this style's capabilities.

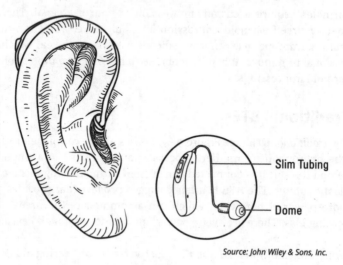

FIGURE 9-5:
Slim tube
hearing aid.
Note: *Like the
traditional BTE, all
components are
encased within the
body of the
hearing aid;
amplified sound
travels through the
slim tubing to the
ear canal.*

Slim Tubing

Dome

Source: John Wiley & Sons, Inc.

Receiver-in-the-canal style

With a newer *receiver-in-the-canal* (RIC) BTE (see Figure 9-6), the receiver or speaker sits in the dome or small earmold in the wearer's ear canal and is connected to the body of the hearing aid behind the ear via a wire. This means that the signal output is being delivered right into the wearer's ear rather than having to travel through tubing from the hearing aid body sitting behind the ear. This style may result in a clearer, crisper signal and can reduce feedback. Its design is smaller and more discrete. The major drawback to this style is that the receiver and wire are delicate and require regular maintenance (see Chapter 11) and a gentle touch to avoid becoming damaged easily.

FIGURE 9-6:
Receiver-in-the-canal hearing aid. **Note:** *In this model, the speaker is now in the dome so amplified sound does not travel through any tubing but rather is delivered directly into the wearer's ear canal.*

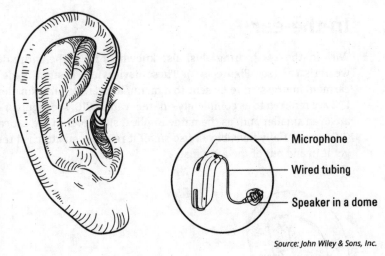

- Microphone
- Wired tubing
- Speaker in a dome

Source: John Wiley & Sons, Inc.

Open and closed styles

Slim tube and RIC styles often use domes rather than custom earmolds for the part that sits in the ear canal. These domes can be open or closed fit, which refers to whether the domes have holes in them (open fit) or not (closed fit). People with milder, high-frequency hearing losses can use open fit domes, which allow for more natural sound to enter the ear canal and allow for the ear canal to breathe. Conversely, closed fit domes are used for more moderate or severe hearing loss as they block outside sound and amplify low-frequency sounds.

TECHNICAL
STUFF

Open domes help prevent the *occlusion effect* — that is, when your ears feel plugged up and your voice sounds louder to you with an echo-like quality. You might also refer to this sound quality as "hollow" or "booming." This happens because when we move our jaw to speak or chew, we create vibrations in the ear canal. When the ear canal is completely blocked with a hearing aid or earmold, those vibrations can't escape and result in the occlusion effect. People who have better low-frequency hearing and use closed domes, earmolds, or ITE-style hearing aids are more likely to report experiencing the occlusion effect. Should you run into this issue, check with your hearing professional. Fun fact: You can simulate the occlusion effect by repeating words and sentences aloud with and without your fingers plugging up your ear canal (alright, maybe not that fun).

In-the-ear

With in-the-ear hearing aids, also known as ITEs, the entire device sits in the wearer's ear (see Figure 9-7). These devices are custom made and require an earmold impression to be sent to a manufacturer. Popular smaller variants of the ITE are referred to as completely-in-the-canal (CIC; see Figure 9-8). These styles are even smaller and, as the name implies, sit deeper in the ear canal. In fact, the CIC is essentially invisible and so small it requires an attached removal handle to get it in and out of the ear canal.

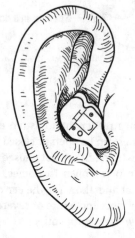

FIGURE 9-7:
In-the-ear
hearing aid.
Note: *The
amplifier and
processor are
encased within the
body of the
hearing aid just
behind the
microphone.*

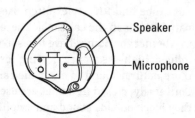

Speaker

Microphone

Source: John Wiley & Sons, Inc.

FIGURE 9-8:
Completely-in-
the-canal
hearing aid.
Note: The
amplifier and
processor are
encased within
the body of the
hearing aid just
behind the
microphone.

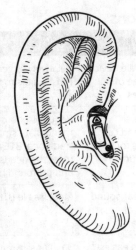
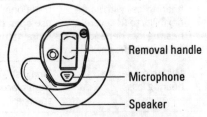

Removal handle
Microphone
Speaker

Source:John Wiley & Sons, Inc.

WARNING

The primary purpose of the CIC is cosmetic. A major drawback is that the small size comes at the expense of power. These small hearing aids are intended for mild hearing loss and cannot address the needs of more moderate or severe loss. The size also limits the features available; CICs often can't use advanced technology features like directionality. Some users who choose these styles become disappointed in their hearing aids and believe them to be ineffective when, in reality, these people have been fit with a hearing aid that is inappropriate for their level of hearing loss or hearing needs.

TIP

ITEs are a great option when the user has problems inserting and manipulating behind-the-ear–style hearing aids due to numbness in their fingers or arthritis. The custom shape of the ITE makes it somewhat easier to slip into the ear.

Weighing the pros and cons of hearing aid styles

Picking the right hearing aid for you requires checking out the pros and cons of each style of hearing aid. Take a look at Table 9-1 to see which style may be the one for you.

TABLE 9-1: Hearing Aid Styles Pros and Cons

Type	Used For	Pros	Cons
Traditional behind-the-ear	All degrees of hearing loss from mild to profound	Extremely versatile device with widest range of available features	Relatively larger in size and most visible to the eye
Slim tube behind-the-ear	Mild to moderate hearing loss with some flexibility to fit severe hearing loss depending on the specific device	Less visible than traditional BTE and can use open domes for more natural sound	Requires enough dexterity to manipulate smaller size than traditional BTE and doesn't meet the needs of most severe and profound hearing losses
Receiver in the canal behind-the-ear	Mild to moderate hearing loss	Smallest BTE, clear sound from placement of speaker in the ear	Most fragile BTE
In-the-ear	Mild to severe hearing loss	Custom fit that is easiest to use when wearer has limited dexterity	Smaller size may limit a few features
Completely in-the-canal	Mild hearing loss	Nearly invisible	Small size limits power and features like directionality

IN THIS CHAPTER

» **Discovering your hearing aid needs**

» **Recognizing the need for two hearing aids**

» **Deciding if prescription hearing aids are the way to go**

» **Finding over-the-counter options**

» **Aligning your lifestyle to your hearing aid**

Chapter **10**

Understanding Your Hearing Aid Options

The thought of navigating the purchase of a hearing aid can be overwhelming — there are hundreds and hundreds of devices to choose from. Many of these come in multiple styles and sizes. Different categories of hearing aids exist, including the new, as of 2022, over-the-counter hearing aid category in the United States.

In this chapter, we explain the two major ways of purchasing hearing aids — over-the-counter and prescription — and we discuss the process of customizing a hearing aid. This chapter gives you the basic foundational knowledge to help guide your decisions when purchasing your own hearing aids.

Discovering Where to Start for Your Needs

Ready to purchase hearing aids? Before jumping right into navigating the hearing aid market, take a minute to reflect on your needs. We break it down into three steps:

1. **Check your hearing.**

   Get a professional diagnostic hearing test (see Chapter 6) or use a smartphone-based hearing test such as the free Mimi or SonicCloud hearing test in your smartphone's app store.

   REMEMBER

   OTC hearing aids are appropriate for mild to moderate hearing loss, while prescription hearing aids can address any degree of hearing loss from mild to profound (see Chapter 7).

2. **Spend some time thinking about your hearing needs.**

   Seriously, take some time to write down the kinds of situations in which you're experiencing difficulty. Think about the details of the situation, the people you're speaking with, the size and layout of the space, competing noise, and any adjustments you've tried so far. Use these situations to create listening goals and think about how those goals fit into your everyday life. Having your goals and lifestyle clearly spelled out ahead of time helps you align your hearing needs to different levels of technology.

3. **Take a moment to think about the type of person you are.**

   How much research are you willing to do? Are you self-motivated or do you need someone else to push you along? If you're already feeling overwhelmed, even after reading this book, then it may be best to start by making an appointment with a professional. If you're a DIY kind of person, look through the information and resources in this book.

Knowing Two Ears Means Two Hearing Aids

Your brain is designed to use sound from two ears (see Chapter 2). In fact, hearing with two ears is much easier than only one ear because it provides the brain extra, redundant information to make sense of sound. In most cases, you want to use two hearing aids to take advantage of our brains' design. The benefits of two hearing aids include these:

>> Requires less amplification to hear softer sounds

>> Makes it easier to localize sounds in the environment

>> Improves clarity and the ability to distinguish sounds, especially in noise

>> Creates a sense of balance and comfort when listening

Is using only one hearing aid harmful?

While using two hearing aids has some clear advantages, is using only one actually bad? The answer is not really. You might become accustomed to using only one hearing aid, which would make it harder to adjust to using two at a later date. Also, you may struggle more if you use only one. But for people with hearing loss that develops over time, except for certain exceptions (see the next section, "The exception to the rule"), there is no evidence that there is anything wrong with only using one hearing aid.

TECHNICAL STUFF

You may encounter websites or professionals saying that using only one hearing aid is actually harmful and can cause *auditory deprivation*, which is the idea that without stimulation, the ear rapidly degrades. These statements are based on several older studies; there is little modern evidence that only wearing one hearing aid is actually harmful.

The exception to the rule

There may be rare cases where one hearing aid is better than two. For people with dementia, cognitive impairment, or auditory processing disorders, it may be easier to use one hearing aid. This could be due to a cognitive issue in processing two signals.

WHAT TO DO WHEN ONE EAR DOESN'T WORK AT ALL

Our brains simply do best with two ears. Most people have hearing loss that is symmetrical in both ears. That is to say, for most people, if they have mild hearing loss in their right ear, they have similarly mild hearing loss in the left ear. But some people have large differences in hearing between their ears. In extreme cases, some people have one ear that essentially has no useable hearing and the other ear has useable hearing with anywhere from normal to severe hearing loss. The technical term for this is *single-sided deafness* or *single-sided hearing loss,* but you may see this referred to as a *dead ear,* which is not a name that we care for but is commonly used.

Adults with single-sided hearing loss require unique solutions and should work with a hearing care professional to find a solution that works for them. While some people

(continued)

(continued)

with single-sided hearing loss do nothing if their good ear has normal hearing or just use one hearing aid if the good ear has some hearing loss, there is another option called the CROS, which stands for Contralateral Routing of Signals.

The CROS system involves wearing two devices that look like hearing aids. The device on the bad ear transmits sound to the good ear. So even though only one ear is listening, that one ear is sending two signals to the brain essentially simulating listening with two ears. Using a CROS system can improve the ability to localize sound, makes listening in noise easier, and helps with hearing and distinguishing softer sounds.

Along with the CROS system, there are also surgical options for treating single-sided hearing loss that are covered in Chapter 13. These include getting a cochlear implant or osseointegrated hearing implant in the affected ear. These types of surgically implantable technologies are very different from each other and from a CROS system. Each option has its own pros and cons that an audiologist and ENT can discuss with you.

Choosing a Prescription Hearing Aid

Prescription hearing aids will continue to operate in the traditional model of hearing care, where hearing aids are purchased through a professional. The only major difference in the technology between prescription and OTC is that prescription hearing aids can meet the needs of people with any degree of hearing loss, including severe and profound hearing loss, whereas the OTC devices are limited to mild and moderate hearing loss.

The prescription hearing aid model is a great option for those with mild to moderate hearing loss who don't want to worry about making decisions themselves or spend time doing their own research. If you want the guidance and involvement of a professional every step of the way, seek out prescription hearing aids. But remember that it may be more costly from the start because you'll be paying for professional services in addition to the price of the hearing aid (see Chapter 15 for more on pricing).

Working with a professional to purchase hearing aids

Researchers and clinicians have spent decades designing a set of best practices to help people with hearing loss benefit from their hearing aids. Hearing professionals, audiologists, and hearing instrument specialists study these best practices to pass onto you during appointments. The process of working with a professional may seem time intensive, but the experience of a professional may save time (and money) in the long run.

REMEMBER

We know we sound like a broken record, but we can't make this point enough. By design, prescription hearing aids are linked to the services of a professional and the costs are often bundled together. But remember, whether you buy an OTC hearing aid or a prescription hearing aid, you can always seek and benefit from the guidance of a professional.

The following sections look at what working with a professional for hearing aids looks like.

The diagnostic hearing test

During a hearing test appointment, your hearing professional will test your hearing using a combination of assessments where you respond to tones or beeps and repeat words and sentences. These test results will help determine your type and degree of hearing loss. See Chapters 6 and 7 for more details on testing.

REMEMBER

For some types of hearing loss, your hearing professional may recommend seeing a physician to rule out any medical causes of hearing loss.

Needs assessment and selecting a hearing aid

The hearing professional will ask you a series of questions about your experience with hearing loss and the types of situations in which you experience difficulties. In addition, you will discuss your lifestyle, including how active you are, your hobbies, your work environment, and people you regularly communicate with. The hearing professional will want to find out as much as possible about your difficulties and your lifestyle to help guide recommendations for a hearing aid brand and technology level.

TIP

Be prepared ahead of time with as many specific details as possible on the trouble you have experienced and in what settings. The more information you provide, the better.

REMEMBER

There is no evidence that a higher cost or level of technology ensures a better result. But some of the features reflected in the level of technology can make addressing certain situations easier or may be preferred depending on your personality type. For example, would you rather have a hearing aid that requires you to manually change the settings by pushing a button or a device that automatically adjusts without you having to think about it? (See the later section, "Choosing Basic or Premium Hearing Aids.")

Customizing your hearing aids with a professional

Once you and your hearing professional decide on a prescription hearing aid, an order will be placed. When the hearing aid comes in, you'll attend a fitting appointment to customize the hearing aids.

HEARING AID FEATURES: TOO MANY TO COUNT

When you're hearing aid shopping, you're going to be bombarded with the names of various features. Here are some of the main ones you'll see and what they mean. But keep in mind that every hearing aid manufacturer uses a slightly different name.

- A **channel** refers to groups of frequencies or pitches that can be independently adjusted. Multiple channels mean a hearing aid can create a highly customized output based on your hearing loss so that you're getting volume where you need it.

- **Directionality** refers to hearing aids' ability to focus on sounds in a specific area around you, usually right in front but it could be any direction, while dampening sounds in other areas.

- **Wind reduction** is a feature that limits the impact of wind blowing over the hearing aid microphone and creating a whistling sensation.

- **Noise reduction or speech enhancement** are broad terms that refer to the hearing aids' processing features that can recognize and enhance people talking while identifying and dampening noise.

- **Feedback suppression** is the hearing aid's ability to limit the whistling or buzzing that occurs when sound escapes and is reamplified by the hearing aid.

- **Wireless connectivity** refers to the device's ability to use Bluetooth or other wireless connections to connect to consumer electronic devices to allow for situations such as streaming a phone call through hearing aids or controlling hearing aids with a smartphone app.

- **Occlusion control** is when the hearing aid uses special sound processing techniques to help make your own voice sound less like an echo or boom.

- **Volume control** is simply the ability to adjust the volume of the hearing aid yourself by using either a button, toggle, or wheel on the hearing aid or with a remote control or smartphone app.

- **Programs** is when a hearing aid can use a combination of specific output settings and some features to make a program setting for a specific listening situation, such as a restaurant or concert.

- **Binaural synchronization** refers to the ability of two hearing aids to work together via a wireless connection, to, for example, adjust just one device to raise the volume of both.

- **Automatic adjustment** is an advanced feature where the hearing aids use cues in your environment to adjust the settings without any user input. This means the hearing aids could switch from a general settings mode to a specialized restaurant setting mode without you needing to do anything.

- **Frequency lowering** is a signal processing feature where the hearing aids move sounds from high to low frequencies to take advantage of better hearing in lower frequencies (remember that most people have high-frequency hearing loss while hearing in low frequencies is normal or near-normal). Most people don't notice the difference, but this can give sound a more bass-like quality.

The hearing aid fitting

During your fitting appointment, the hearing professional will connect the hearing aid to a computer and enter your test results to produce a custom prescription for your type and degree of hearing loss. In addition, the hearing professional may create some programs in the hearing aid to address very specific situations you described during your needs assessment. These can be relatively universal programs like for a noisy restaurant situation where the hearing aid focuses on what is in front of you and dampens other ambient sounds or an outdoor activity program like running that engages in stronger wind reduction. Alternatively, these programs can be highly customized by the professional for your specific needs, like a program that overemphasizes high-frequency sounds for listening to birds in your backyard or something specifically designed for office meetings.

TECHNICAL STUFF

After initial programming of the hearing aid is complete, best practice dictates the use of a technique called *real ear measurement*. In short, real ear measurement is a process that verifies whether the hearing aid is doing what we expect it to do. Discrepancies can occur because the hearing aid sits differently in your ear canal than the equipment used to test hearing. A small microphone is placed in the ear canal at the same time as the hearing aid is inserted into the ear. Then various sound clips are played. The real ear measurement microphone tells us how much amplification the hearing aid is adding and whether it is the correct amount for your specific needs.

Adjustments are made to ensure the hearing aid is meeting prescriptive targets. Without this process, the hearing professional doesn't know whether your hearing aid is doing what it should be or not.

TIP

Real ear measures are a vital aspect of best-practice hearing care when using a prescription hearing aid. Always ask whether your hearing care professional routinely performs them. Some OTC hearing aids would benefit from real ear measurement as well. If you're feeling like your OTC hearing aid isn't meeting your needs, you may want to consult with a hearing care professional.

Following the hearing aid programming, the hearing professional will sit down with you and walk you through daily use and maintenance, including

>> Inserting and removing your hearing aids

>> Cleaning your hearing aids

>> Changing or recharging the batteries

>> Adjusting the hearing aids if there is a manual volume or program control

Lastly, a good hearing professional will dedicate lots of time to setting realistic goals and creating the right expectations for hearing aid use. Remember, no matter how good the hearing aids, you'll need to take the time to get used to them, and your hearing won't be perfect. See Chapter 11 for more information on expectations.

Follow-up appointments

Most professionals will want to see you back in a few weeks to discuss your experience with your hearing aids and review information covered during the first fitting appointment (it's a lot to take in all at once!). At follow-up appointments, hearing professionals use a combination of programming adjustments to the hearing aid and counseling to address any concerns you have.

In the initial months following the first fitting appointment, you can expect to see your hearing care professional fairly regularly — at least four appointments in the first six months. Once you and your hearing care professional feel good about where you are with your hearing aid journey, you will likely move on to appointments every six months to check in, adjust if needed, and allow the hearing care professional a chance to check the hearing aids for any wear and tear.

TIP

We think a sign of good hearing care professionals is that they continuously revisit your personal listening goals and set new goals based on your changing lifestyle.

Warranties and insurance

Most prescription hearing aids come with a two- or three-year service warranty that covers any malfunctions or necessary repairs. In addition, there's usually a one-time per hearing aid loss and damage replacement warranty. This means that the manufacturer will replace each hearing aid one time if it is lost or damaged beyond repair during the warranty period.

Many hearing care professionals work with insurance companies that offer extended repair and replacement warranties beyond the initial manufacturer warranty. It is always a good idea to ask your hearing care professional about these options before the initial warranty expires.

Warranties among OTC hearing aids may vary from company to company in scope and length of time.

Navigating the Over-the-Counter Hearing Aid Pathway

Over-the-counter (OTC) hearing aids, expected to become available by late 2022, create a new accessible and affordable category of hearing aids. Individuals will no longer need to consult a professional to purchase hearing aids, which makes getting OTC hearing aids a more rapid process (although you may still want to consult a professional before or after your purchase).

REMEMBER

As this book goes to press, the over-the-counter hearing aid marketplace is only just taking shape. We don't have all the answers, but let's walk through some considerations for what navigating the pathway might look like.

The basics of OTC hearing aids

The media have been covering OTC hearing aids since the first reports of the OTC Hearing Aid Act was in Congress in 2017. It can be confusing to try to dig through the various reports on OTC hearing aids to really understand the differences between OTC hearing aids and prescription hearing aids. And it is downright impossible to read the U.S. Food and Drug Administration (FDA) documents on OTC hearing aids (well, not impossible, but *definitely* not easy or enjoyable). Fortunately, we're here to walk through the basics of OTC hearing aids together.

Who are OTC hearing aids for?

Over-the-counter hearing aids are intended for adults with mild to moderate hearing loss. While there are no other requirements, it's worth noting that many OTC options may require some familiarity with using a smartphone to initially set up the devices, so keep that in mind if considering this option.

THE UNEVEN AND CHANGING HEARING AID LANDSCAPE OF THE UNITED STATES

In the United States, hearing aids are medical devices regulated by the U.S. Food and Drug Administration (FDA), which broadly defines hearing aids as wearable instruments or devices that are intended to treat hearing loss. Since the 1970s, FDA-approved hearing aids could be sold only through licensed professionals. The initial hearing aid technology was useless if it wasn't programmed by a trained professional.

While this model of care has successfully met the needs of some individuals with hearing loss, many Americans simply can't afford or access hearing aids. Less than 20 to 30 percent of Americans with hearing loss own and use hearing aids. While not every single individual with hearing loss needs hearing aids, there are clearly millions of additional individuals with hearing loss who would benefit from hearing aids. Published research shows that from 2011 to 2018, hearing aid use increased 30 percent among the wealthiest older Americans, while those at or below the poverty line saw an overall 13 percent decrease in hearing aid ownership.

The need for change was not lost on those who were paying attention. In August 2017, the U.S. Congress passed the bipartisan Over-the-Counter Hearing Aid Act, instructing the FDA to create an over-the-counter (OTC) category of hearing aids to allow for increased consumer access to affordable hearing aids. In November 2021, the FDA proposed draft regulations for OTC hearing aids that are slated to go into effect in late 2022.

TECHNICAL STUFF

Wondering why OTC hearing aids aren't for all degrees of hearing loss? It's a safety concern. More severe hearing losses require a lot of volume to address. Because no professional will be involved in the process, there will be limitations on how loud OTC hearing aids can make sound to ensure the devices don't damage anyone's hearing.

TIP

The new category of OTC hearing aids may be especially useful for those who noticed trouble hearing in only one or two very specific situations but never felt the cost and time required to get conventional prescription hearing aids was worth it. With their lower price point and easy access, OTC hearing aids may fill this gap by offering a readily available and affordable option.

Meeting minimum government standards

You may see people describe OTC hearing aids as "deregulation," but this couldn't be further from the truth. The FDA will hold OTC hearing aids to strict technical standards to ensure higher quality devices that can meet the needs of adults with mild to moderate hearing loss. In fact, a happy little side effect of the OTC hearing aid category is that for the first time in decades, many hearing aid companies will be forced to perform clinical studies to provide evidence that their hearing aids meet the minimum standards.

This is great for, you, the consumer, as you can look for the label of FDA-approved OTC hearing aids as a sign of reassurance that these devices meet technical specifications to ensure the devices are safe and effective.

Purchasing without a professional

Over the counter means these devices will be available without going through a professional.

With prescription hearing aids, the price that a consumer pays for the hearing aids often accounts for both the cost of the hearing aids bundled together with the costs of the professional services to fit and program the devices and provide education and counseling to the patient. With the imminent availability of OTC hearing aids, consumers will soon be able to purchase just the hearing aids without these other professional hearing care services being bundled in automatically, allowing for greater price transparency. This is a good thing for everyone!

To use a car analogy: Hearing professionals may soon go from being seen as "car salespersons," mostly focused on sales of hearing aids, to "mechanics," who offer support services such as care and maintenance. Obviously, there is more to it than that, but getting rid of the "sales focused" perception that many people have about hearing care professionals is great!

TIP

As we've said, just because OTC hearing aids are not sold through hearing professionals doesn't mean you can't consult them. If you're struggling to decide on OTC options, it may be worth consulting a professional to discuss the best options for addressing your hearing needs. And you can consult a professional after buying an OTC hearing aid for help adjusting or troubleshooting the device. In the past, many hearing care professionals wouldn't necessarily offer such services unless you bought a hearing aid from them, but we expect this will rapidly change as OTC hearing aids come to market. *Note:* These professional hearing care services will often not be covered by insurance. Check your policy; you may have to pay out of pocket.

Limitless possibilities

Over-the-counter hearing aids are just getting started and could take on many shapes, sizes, and designs. Some will look similar to wireless earbuds, while others will take the route of more traditional behind-the-ear hearing aid designs.

Adjusting the devices will also vary from company to company. Some will be customizable by integrating with smartphone apps that can do a hearing test to precisely program the OTC hearing aid. Others may use various preset programs that the user can scroll through with a push button and volume control.

We expect the category of OTC hearing aids will modernize the hearing aid market in the United States and make it easier for adults to get hearing aids. Competition from companies entering the hearing aid market will drive down pricing and spur new technologic advances. It's a very exciting time for hearing aids in the United States, and we can't wait to see what the future brings.

If you've got mild to moderate hearing loss and you're a self-motivated, do-it-yourself kind of person or just someone who wants to try a lower-cost hearing aid, OTC hearing aids may be the place to start. You can always consult a professional later to obtain hearing care services or look into prescription hearing aids.

Deciding where to buy your OTC hearing aid

Over-the-counter hearing aids will be on store shelves and online. Each option comes with pros and cons depending on your needs and desires. To check on pricing and payment options, turn to Chapter 15.

At the store

Stores that sell OTC hearing aids could range from pharmacies like CVS and Walgreens to technology outlets like Best Buy and large box stores like Costco, Sam's Club, and Walmart. Making a purchase in-person allows you to get a feel for the true size and shape of the device.

Purchasing in a store may also come with the added benefit of an additional store warranty or some help from the professionals who staff the store. For example, Best Buy has the Geek Squad, a team of technology professionals to help troubleshoot options and may be able to assist with device purchases. Big box stores like Sam's Club and Costco already employ hearing professionals in many locations to sell prescription hearing aids. In the future, we could see those professionals integrating options to support OTC hearing aids.

Purchasing online

Online retailers offer a streamlined process with just the click of a few buttons. You'll be able to read reviews from other users that can help guide decision-making. The websites or apps may even integrate online hearing testing options or questionnaires to help guide purchases based on lifestyle and degree of hearing loss.

How to choose from too many options

The new OTC hearing aid category will allow for numerous new companies to produce hearing aids. Increasing competition is great for cost and for innovation, but it can be hard to navigate all those options. When considering OTC hearing aids, some of the following points may help with your decision.

Self-programming

Pay attention to how the device is programmed and whether it allows the user to make changes to the sound output. You want to look for devices that allow you to customize for your hearing loss and further fine-tune settings like a volume control to make preferential changes. There are many ways to customize an OTC hearing aid, including through preset programs, smartphone integration, or a way to enter results from a hearing test.

TIP

A great way to ensure a good fit is to look for devices that are integrated with a smartphone. Ideally, the OTC hearing aids' smartphone app will allow you to test your hearing while wearing the OTC hearing aids to customize the output of the device. This process can result in some of the best hearing aid fittings that resemble the prescription hearing aids fine-tuned by a professional.

TECHNICAL STUFF

Why is the process of doing a hearing test through the OTC hearing aid so valuable? Using different devices in the ear for a hearing test versus the actual hearing aid can cause some mismatches that result in a poorer hearing aid customization. This is because different devices sit differently in the ear canal, and just a small change in the way a product fits in the ear can have a huge effect on sound output. In the clinical setting, professionals work to correct these differences. OTC hearing aids that perform testing through the product itself can overcome this issue.

Warranties and support

A good rule of thumb is always to look for OTC hearing aid companies that stand behind their brand. A warranty or money-back return period after purchase can offer some level of reassurance before purchasing. Some companies may go the extra step of also offering online or phone support, options for mail-in support for damages and repairs, or a recommended network of professionals who can support the company's device.

Look for features and programs

Seeing how features align with your lifestyle can help guide your purchase decisions. If you plan to use the hearing aid in many different settings, for instance, it will be useful to look for devices that specifically advertise features and programs for different situations.

Hearing aid programs combine several features to optimize hearing in specific settings. Some common special programs are "calm," "restaurant," and "music" settings. For example, restaurant settings will use directionality and noise reduction features to focus on speakers in front of you and aggressively reduce ambient noise (see Chapter 9), while calm settings focus on sound from all directions and amplify any sound around you. Music settings tend to do as little manipulation as possible to present the music in the way it was meant to be heard and avoid the hearing aid dampening sounds that are intended to be loud or sharp.

Conversely, if you don't plan to use the hearing aids in a variety of settings, you may not need any extra features or programs. One standard setting with a volume wheel may do the trick.

When to seek professional assistance with OTC hearing aids

Audiologists, who hold a doctoral degree in measuring and treating hearing loss, and hearing instrument specialists, who focus exclusively on selling and fitting hearing aids, can play a key role in supporting OTC hearing aids. Leveraging their experience and expertise can be helpful when you're in need of assistance.

There are many situations when professional guidance may be helpful:

>> You feel like you should be doing better with the OTC hearing aids.

>> You just can't seem to get your OTC hearing aid to work in specific situations.

>> You noticed a change in either your hearing or in the output of the device.

>> Your OTC hearing aid stops functioning.

>> You initially purchased the OTC hearing aid to help with only one or two specific situations but now notice you've been missing out on other situations. You'd like to try other options but aren't sure where to start.

The general rule is that if you have consulted the manual or other support options from the OTC hearing aid manufacturer but still feel frustrated or find your hearing aids aren't meeting your needs, then schedule an appointment with a professional.

The hearing care professional may ask you questions about your experience, test your hearing, and examine your OTC hearing aid. The professional may offer counseling to set appropriate expectations, give advice on adjusting the OTC hearing aid, or demonstrate maintenance procedures on the OTC hearing aid.

REMEMBER

Hearing professionals may also find your hearing aid isn't right for you and recommend a different product based on your hearing test results and needs.

A few things to check before making an appointment with a hearing care professional:

TIP

>> **Be clear about what you want.** Make sure the hearing aid professional knows why you're coming in for an appointment.

>> **Make sure that professional works with all types of hearing aids.** Some professionals work in hearing aid clinics that are owned by specific hearing aid manufacturers and only work with specific brands of hearing aids.

>> **Ask for rates ahead of time.** Not all hearing care professionals have clear hourly rates for providing such hearing care services, as some may only provide these services bundled into the purchase of a hearing aid.

Choosing Basic or Premium Hearing Aids

When navigating the hearing aid marketplace, whether prescription or OTC, you may see terms like "basic" and "premium" technology. In fact, you'll often see the same hearing aid name with multiple versions. As a hypothetical, you might see a product called the "Dummies Hearing Aid" in four versions: The Dummies Hearing Aid 100, 200, 300, and 400. The numbers at the end refer to the level of technology (100 would be basic, while 400 would be top of the line).

The technology level usually has little to do with the hardware but rather the software in the hearing aid that allows for more advanced automated features and signal processing. For example, basic hearing aids will usually have the directionality feature (a fixed focus on sound right in front of a user while dampening sound behind the user), but it requires the user to turn directionality on and off by pressing a button. The premium version of that same hearing aid may have the ability to automatically switch to directionality mode without the user's input in certain environments (for example, a noisy restaurant) without requiring the user to do anything. Rather than being fixed only on what is in front of the user, the area of focus can change according to where people are speaking. This could be very useful in an environment with several speakers.

Each hearing aid manufacturer prices and groups the features differently. When selecting a hearing aid and choosing between different levels of technology, a good guide is to use your lifestyle and personality type to choose the technology. Are you in a lot of varied listening environments and want to be able to set the hearing aid once and not worry about having to adjust to different environments? Then maybe more premium technology is worthwhile for you. But you can be just as successful with basic technology.

Audiologists and hearing aid specialists hate when we use this analogy, but we like to think of basic and premium technology just like cars. Many manufacturers have an economy and a luxury brand. Is it nice to ride in a car with heated leather seats, cruise control, and a high-tech dash display? Sure. But will an economy class car also get you from point A to point B? Yes, it will. Moreover, both car levels require the same care and upkeep to maintain the vehicle, and sometimes it's not the car but a special accessory that gets you through tough situations (think snow tires).

We view hearing aids the same way: All levels have the potential to get you to where you need to be and still require the same customization and maintenance. The difference is in the journey. Take the example of a big family dinner. A basic hearing aid can be customized to the output you need and offers the ability to manually turn on directionality mode that focuses on sounds right in front of you, so you get a little boost of what you're looking at. This means that you have to turn your head and look at the sound you want to hear. After dinner, you might join the family to listen to some music, so you turn off the directionality mode and manually activate a music mode. A premium hearing aid with automatic adjustments would pick up the sound in the room and turn directionality mode on and off without you needing to lift a finger. Premium devices could also adjust the directionality focus without you needing to turn your head, so if someone directly to your right is speaking, the hearing aids will focus there. Then premium aids would automatically enter a music mode after dinner without you needing to think about it. Perhaps during dinner, regardless of basic or premium technology, you also use a special accessory called a remote mic (see Chapter 12), which significantly helps in noisy situations and makes all the difference. Just like the cars example, both basic and premium tech get you through the night, but one is likely just a smoother experience.

REMEMBER

Researchers at the University of Memphis compared premium and basic devices to assess hearing-related outcomes such as understanding speech. They found no difference. The authors of the study concluded that it shouldn't be assumed that higher levels of technology or more costly hearing aids will always produce better results. An important thing to remember is that in that study, all the participants had access to an audiologist who followed best-practice guidelines, which the researchers emphasized was more important than the device technology level or cost.

Chapter **11**

You've Got Hearing Aids: Now What?

You got your hearing tested and used the test results to select and purchase new hearing aids. Congratulations! You're done now, right? Not so much. Hearing care is a journey that doesn't end with acquiring the hearing aids. Entering this next step of your journey with the right expectations and knowledge can make all the difference in hearing aid success. We think your attitude and actions are so important that we've ordered this chapter to start there.

In this chapter, we're honest with you about what you should expect with hearing aid use. A hearing aid is not a magic pill. We share with you activities you can do to train your brain to use your hearing aids and take a deep dive into the care and maintenance routines that can help you maximize the lifespan of your hearing aids. Most people love their hearing aids, and in this chapter we show you the steps to take so you can, too.

Setting Expectations Is Key

Having the right mindset and setting realistic expectations from the start will set you up for success. We've seen clients who set their expectations too high face disappointment.

Let's start with a cold, hard fact about hearing aid use. Hearing aids will not "correct" hearing. We lose our hearing when cellular damage occurs in the cochlea or inner ear that limits our ability to detect sounds in our environment (see Chapter 3 for more detail). Hearing aids are amazing pieces of technology that augment and manipulate sound to address hearing loss, but in the end, hearing aids are just "aids" that will never truly replace normal hearing.

This is quite in contrast to eyeglasses, which for most forms of vision loss correct your vision. Not so with hearing aids. Nonetheless, the majority of hearing aid users are successful. Following are some key expectations for success:

>> **Expect to put in effort.** Consider training for a 5K run. When you first start training, you start slow and short. You may tire fast and feel sore after every practice run. Over time, you build up strength and endurance, and eventually, you reach a point where running a 5K is just second nature. Similarly, the most successful hearing aid users practice using different settings and wear their hearing aids as often as possible. That effort pays dividends over time as you adjust to your hearing aids and find out what works best for you.

>> **Expect to focus on narrow situations rather than overall hearing.** Listening to your family talk in a restaurant is different from listening to music on the car radio. Shifting your mindset from setting broad goals like "hearing better" to very specific situational goals like "listening to my friend tell a story at our favorite restaurant over lunch" goes a long way. Narrowing your expectations to a specific situation creates an achievable goal where you can find the right combination of hearing aid settings, communication tips (see Chapter 8), and assistive devices (see Chapter 12) to improve that situation.

>> **Expect a hearing care journey.** Give your brain time to adjust to your new hearing aids, to any new adjustments your professional makes, and to each new situation you find yourself in. The hearing care journey never stops. Creating routines and habits makes hearing aid use second nature.

TIP

If you're working with a professional, expect that to be a long-term relationship with frequent visits as you start off and then at least two visits a year. You will want to find someone you are compatible with and will want to continue working with for the long run.

>> **Expect better but not flawless results.** As we note earlier, hearing aids don't correct hearing. A healthy mindset is to expect to improve your current hearing, but not to deceive yourself into thinking everything will be perfect.

>> **Expect a unique experience.** No two people have the exact same hearing aid journey. What works for someone else may not work for you and vice versa. Don't compare your journey to others. Instead, stay focused on your own plan and goals.

REMEMBER

If your hearing test showed you have trouble understanding speech (see Chapter 7), you may still struggle even when using hearing aids. Consider this when setting your expectations and make sure you talk to a hearing care professional about all your options.

Getting Used to Your Hearing Aids

Some people expect hearing aids to instantly return everything to their perception of normal with perfect clarity. Of course, we know you will know better and set appropriate expectations because you've read this chapter!

REMEMBER

The reality is that hearing aid use is a journey, and it takes time to get used to your new hearing aids. When you put in your new hearing aids, you'll hear sounds you haven't fully heard for a long time, and they may not sound the way you remember them or the sounds are different from what you've gotten used to. It can be slightly unsettling when something you hear every day, like your own voice, suddenly sounds different.

Hearing loss sets in at a slow pace. In fact, it's so slow that we hardly notice hearing loss at first. We don't know what we're missing. Most people live with some degree of hearing loss for several years before getting hearing aids. During that time, the parts of the ear and brain that would normally detect and process sounds remain inactive. When you get hearing aids, those parts of the ear and brain become active again and can be overstimulated after sitting inactive for so long. This can be a jarring process.

TIP

It helps to think of your ears and brain like muscles. Imagine that you used to lift weights at the gym every day but then took a five-year break and barely exercised. If you returned to the gym and tried to lift the same amount of weight, it would be very difficult! The good news is that with the right routine, you can get back into shape. The same can be said for hearing aid use. With time and dedication, you can get to where you need to be.

Practice makes perfect

The best way to get used to your hearing aids may be obvious: Wear them. The more time you spend listening with your hearing aids, the more you get used to them.

REMEMBER

Hearing aids do a lot to make sounds, particularly speech, easier for you to hear, but those sounds might sound just slightly different from what you used to hear. For example, depending on the wearer's hearing loss, the "s" sound in "snake" may have a more bass-like quality than the high-frequency hissing sound we're used to. Your brain needs time to learn to put these new sounds together and use the output from the hearing aid. You can speed up that process by using hearing aids as often as possible and in as many situations as possible. This includes wearing the hearing aids at home when you think you may not need them.

TIP

Don't avoid situations because you're worried about listening with your new hearing aids. Instead, try to reframe your mindset that you need to practice using your hearing aids in different situations and expect some bumps in the road.

TIP

Try to practice mindful listening with your hearing aids. That is, take time to pay attention to your immediate surroundings. Focus and identify each sound you perceive with your hearing aids. Look for the source of each sound and consciously associate that sound with that source. For example, if you hear whistling, look around and find where it is coming from. It may be a bird. Focus on the sound for a minute and consciously associate the sound you hear with that bird. Taking time to be mindful can help retrain your brain faster.

REMEMBER

While it's best to get as much practice in as possible, don't forget to also enjoy some silence and allow your brain time to relax. You can try the same mindfulness technique with you hearing aids on in a quiet room and just focus on your breathing and the silence in the room. Relax and enjoy some quiet time. Just like with physical exercise, your ears and brain need recovery periods.

Activities to get used to hearing aids

In addition to wearing your hearing aids throughout the day, it's a great idea to try listening activities with your hearing aids. The following activities, with your hearing aids in, can help you train your brain:

>> **Listen to people with and without background noise.** Have a conversation with someone or watch a TV program with plenty of talking, such as a news program. Then introduce background noise by playing the radio, a podcast, or an audiobook. Start the background noise soft but gradually increase the volume. Keep focusing on the conversation or TV show.

TIP

The visual cues of watching people speak make it easier to understand them. As you get used to your hearing aids, make this activity more difficult by focusing on listening to audio without visual cues — using radio, podcasts, or audiobooks — with background noise.

>> **Read out loud.** We hear our own voices daily. But have you ever heard your voice recorded and played back to you and just hate it? This is because unlike other sounds, we hear our own voice internally through bone conduction (see Chapter 7), which gives it a different quality. When it's played to us via a recording, it sounds different. Similarly, hearing aids may give your voice a different sound. Read aloud to yourself to get used to hearing your own voice with hearing aids.

>> **Get a communication buddy.** Have a friend or family member you feel comfortable with serve as your communication buddy and plan communication outings. Any setting will do (for example, restaurants, outdoor plazas, stores, parks, or concerts). Spend time describing to each other what you hear. Be open with your communication buddy about what you can and cannot clearly hear and try making adjustments like getting closer to the sound, increasing or decreasing the volume of the hearing aid, or activating different hearing aid programs to improve your ability to hear sounds.

>> **Listen to audiobooks.** As you listen, follow along in the print or e-book. Later, only listen to the audiobook. Try to listen to each word carefully and when you struggle, refer to the text.

TIP

Keep track of any speech sounds you have trouble hearing. For example, many people have trouble with soft, high-frequency sounds like the "s" in "snake." This list can help a hearing care professional further fine-tune your hearing aids.

>> **Practice localizing sound.** Find a space either outside or in a large room. Close your eyes and have someone move around and talk to you. Try to guess where they are in relation to you. Add some background noise like the radio or TV to make this task more difficult.

>> **Use a listening program or auditory training program.** Find programs at the Hearing Loss Association of America website such as LACE (Listening and Communication Enhancement) at www.hearingloss.org/hearing-help/ technology/auditory-rehab-programs/. These online programs (some free, some not) use auditory games and activities such as matching sounds to pictures or deciphering purposefully difficult speech to strengthen your brain's listening capabilities. Heads up: Some of these programs advertise they can improve cognition — we're not here to comment on that and are only recommending them for auditory training.

>> **Keep a listening or hearing journal.** Reflect on your listening experiences (including these activities) and consider ways to improve listening in the future. Use this journal to guide adjusting and fine-tuning hearing aids (either with your hearing care professional or by yourself with an OTC hearing aid).

Trust the process

It takes time to get used to hearing aids, and some days will be better than others. This means there will be days where it feels like you took a step backward rather than forward. Keep working at it! There will also be days where it feels like you made a giant leap forward.

WARNING

You may experience a phenomenon referred to as auditory fatigue. This is when listening with hearing loss makes you tired because it takes extra brain effort to process and make sense of sound. Early on, when you're adjusting to the sound of your new hearing aids, you may experience some auditory fatigue from your brain being bombarded by new sound. Don't fret; this is normal. The important thing is to take listening breaks by finding a calm, quiet environment when needed and keep going when you're ready.

Part of the process in getting used to your hearing aids is also trusting the hearing aid programming enough to give it a chance. You'll have to get accustomed to the adjustments you make for different settings. Whether you do it yourself with your OTC hearing aids (see Chapter 10) or work with a hearing care professional, be patient with yourself. This is especially important early on when you're just getting used to your hearing aids.

REMEMBER

It's impossible to predict exactly how you will react or how long it will take to get used to hearing aids because no two experiences are exactly the same. It can take anywhere from a few weeks to nearly six months to get used to hearing aids. Instead of focusing too much on a specific time frame, remember that this is a journey and instead focus on the day-by-day progress you're making.

TIP

When you first start with hearing aids, try not to fiddle with them too much when performing listening exercises. It's important to get used to hearing sounds. This can be especially problematic if your instinct is to keep turning down the volume rather than getting used to appropriate amplified listening levels. Some hearing care professionals may initially disable any volume or programming controls on your hearing aids to prevent you from being tempted to make adjustments rather than get used to your new hearing aids.

Adjusting and Manipulating Your Hearing Aids

From dealing with batteries and inserting your hearing aids to adjusting the sound when needed, you need to be familiar with how to use your hearing aids.

Working with batteries

One of the first things to learn is how to turn on your hearing aids. Hearing aids with disposable batteries turn on and off by opening and closing the battery door, while those with rechargeable batteries usually require you to press and hold a button on the hearing aid itself.

Traditionally, hearing aids used a disposable zinc air battery that lasts anywhere from 3 to 14 days depending on size, the type of hearing aid, and how many hours a day the hearing aid is used. A battery door opens at the bottom of the hearing aid (see Figure 11-1) to allow for changing batteries. Usually, a warning signal will alert you to a pending need for a battery change several hours in advance. None-theless, it is recommended that you carry a backup set of batteries just in case you're out and about.

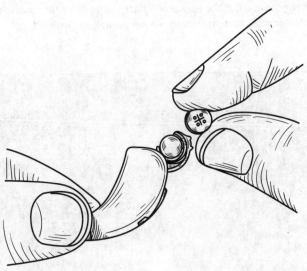

FIGURE 11-1:
The hearing aid battery door.

Source: John Wiley & Sons, Inc.

Newer hearing aids are increasingly turning to rechargeable batteries. These require the user to put the hearing aids on a recharging station every night to have enough juice to get through the next day.

TIP

Aside from eliminating the inconvenience of making regular battery purchases, a major benefit of rechargeable hearing aids is that they are much easier to manip-ulate for adults with dexterity concerns such as arthritis or numbness in their fingers.

Putting hearing aids in your ears

Hearing aids come in different shapes and sizes (check out Chapter 9). Each style requires a different technique to put the hearing aid in your ear. Consult the manual of your hearing aid and talk to your hearing care professional about specific details for your devices.

Here are some general tips and guidelines:

>> Practice inserting and removing your hearing aids with a mirror or friend until it's easy to do.

>> Ask your hearing care professional if you can take a video with a smartphone of a demonstration for inserting and removing the hearing aids in your ears.

>> Try using the hand opposite the hearing aid ear to reach around the back of your ear and pull the ear up and back to open the ear canal while inserting the earmold or dome with the other hand (see Figure 11-2).

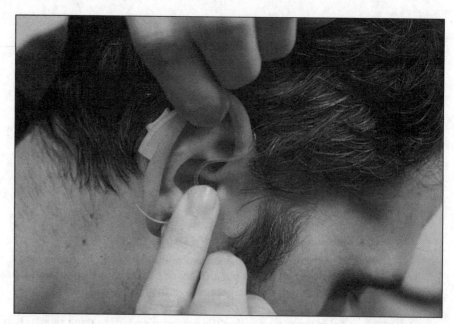

FIGURE 11-2:
Pulling the ear back with your opposite hand and inserting with your other.

Source: Jamie Trumbo, photographer

>> Your hearing aid should fit snugly in your ear, especially if you have a custom earmold. If it is too loose, you may experience whistling and buzzing known as feedback.

>> If you have a behind-the-ear style hearing aid, the wire or tube connecting the body of the hearing aid behind your ear to the dome or earmold in your ear canal should sit tightly up against your skin.

TIP

A research group from the National Health System of the United Kingdom created a series of helpful videos supporting daily hearing aid use, including how to insert hearing aids. We highly recommend giving it a watch: c2hearonline.com/openfit/insertion.html.

Changing the sound of hearing aids

Whether you're using OTC or prescription hearing aids, you usually have some options to adjust your hearing aids. This can help you make changes as needed as you go throughout your day through various listening environments.

With many hearing aids, you can control volume and cycle through various programs for different listening situations. Because of the wide variety of manufacturers, consult your hearing aid manual or hearing care professional for specific details on your device.

In general, there are two main ways to adjust hearing aids:

>> Buttons or switches are located on the back of the hearing aid. This type of hearing aid requires the user to press the button or toggle the switch to control volume or cycle through programs (see Figure 11-3). Many hearing aids alert the user by beeping to indicate that a change has been made. Some hearing aids have settings; for example, pressing a button on the right hearing aid increases the volume while pressing a button on the left hearing aid decreases the volume.

>> Many modern hearing aids, especially those with Bluetooth settings, have remote controls or smartphone apps to adjust the volume or program settings. The use of remote controls or smartphone apps can be easier for those with dexterity issues and usually are more clearly labeled. The hearing aids often alert the user to a change in volume or setting by beeping.

REMEMBER

Some hearing aids have separate volume controls for bass (low frequency) and treble (high frequency). Bass sounds tend to sound louder than treble sounds, so turning up the bass often feels like volume is increasing overall, whereas turning up treble is sometimes barely noticeable. But too much bass can be a bad thing as the low-frequency sounds can overpower the high-frequency sounds. Most hearing loss occurs in higher frequencies; therefore, most people actually need more treble, which adds clarity, than bass volume. Don't overdo it with the bass.

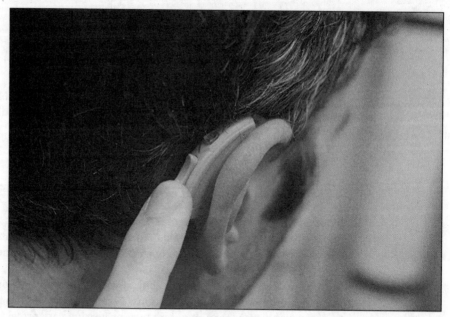

FIGURE 11-3:
Image of a toggle
switch on a
hearing aid.

Source: Jamie Trumbo, photographer

Caring for and Maintaining Your Hearing Aids

Hearing aids are electronic devices that spend most of their time in the ear canal, which is a damp and warm environment. Not exactly the kind of place we expect electronic devices to thrive. In fact, it's basically a hostile environment for hearing aids. Hearing aids aren't necessarily delicate, but like all technology, they're susceptible to wear and tear. You've made a huge investment of your time and money; take care of them. Following some simple routine care practices can make a huge difference in the lifespan of a hearing aid.

Establishing a maintenance routine

Having a daily routine is key. Just like keeping a house tidy, it's significantly easier to straighten up at the end of each day rather than wait until a major deep cleaning is necessary.

Storage

One of the first steps in creating a good maintenance routine is having a single place for hearing aid storage in your home, such as a secure box or hearing aid dryer or dehumidifier on a nightstand or dresser, and a single place for hearing aid storage when you're on the go, usually a small container. Select somewhere indoors that's cool and dry and out of the reach of pets and small children.

Whether this is overnight storage or just intermittent storage throughout the day when you're not planning to wear the hearing aids, keep these places consistent. Honestly, Nick, who has seen many a client's hearing aid go missing, is shouting as he writes this sentence: **Your hearing aids should always be in one of three places: in your ears, in your home storage location, or in your to-go storage location.** Otherwise, you risk misplacing your hearing aids or leaving them somewhere they are vulnerable to damage from water, heat, or pets.

REMEMBER

Always open your battery door when you take your hearing aids out of your ears for storage.

Keeping your hearing aids dry

Moisture is the enemy of any electronic device. Purchasing a hearing aid dryer or dehumidifier is an investment that can pay for itself in years added to the life of a hearing aid. There are two main types of hearing aid dryers: drying jars and electronic dryers.

The jars use capsules with silica beads or gel that wicks away moisture. Simply place the hearing aid in the jar and seal the lid. Usually, the capsules will change colors once the silica beads can no longer absorb any moisture, at which time a new capsule is needed. Typically hearing aids are kept in the jar overnight or as long as possible (any time is better than nothing!).

Alternatively, the electronic dryers, which are more expensive, use air circulation and temperature control to suck away moisture. Often, the electronic dryers have an ultraviolet light system to sterilize the hearing aids as well. Electronic dryers are faster than the dehumidifier and can go through a drying cycle in as little as 30 minutes, but this varies product to product.

Either choice is fine. The important thing is that a daily hearing aid care routine needs to include drying hearing aids every night.

TIP

For rechargeable hearing aids that charge overnight, you can find large hearing aid dryers that the entire charging station can fit inside. If you can't find a dryer that works for your charging setup, create a routine that allows for nightly hearing aid charging as well as time spent in the dryer. This could be placing your hearing aids on the charger when you go to bed and then into the dryer when you wake up while you get ready in the morning. An electronic dryer, which is faster, might be the best option for this setup, but any time in a dryer is better than nothing.

Cleaning

Most hearing aids come with a cleaning kit that includes a small brush with soft bristles, a pick to remove wax, and a microfiber cloth.

Hearing aids should be cleaned daily. The best time to clean them is in the morning, after the hearing aid and all the wax on it have dried out from a night spent in the dryer. Moist wax is difficult to remove. In fact, trying to clean moist wax sometimes just pushes and spreads the wax around, which results in wax getting into places you don't want it — like the microphone or speaker ports.

To clean your hearing aid, hold it gently and first use the soft-bristle brush to clean the entire surface. Then pay close attention to the microphone and the end of the hearing aid that goes into the ear canal. Chapter 9 shows where these generally are on a hearing aid. Alternatively, ask your hearing professional or check your manual for location. Brush over these areas to clean the wax and debris that tend to build up around them — particularly the part that spends time in the ear canal. Open the battery door, if applicable, and brush inside it. Use a gentle back-and-forth motion to clean without any force or pressure. The bristles should touch the hearing aid, but they should not be forcibly bent from pressure.

Most of the dried wax should come off with a good brushing, but you may need a pick to remove pieces that are lodged in any openings around the microphone, speaker, or earmold or dome. Again, use caution and be gentle. Do not try to push the pick into the device.

After brushing and using the pick, give the hearing aid a full wipe-down with the microfiber cloth to remove any remaining wax or debris.

TIP

Get a magnifying glass for giving the hearing aid a good once-over before and after cleaning to make sure you didn't miss any hard-to-see wax or debris.

Things to avoid while cleaning hearing aids

Stick to the provided cleaning kit that came with your hearing aid, if possible. If you're assembling a cleaning kit on your own, only use a soft-bristle brush, microfiber cloth, and products specifically labeled for hearing aid use.

Never use water or household cleaning products to clean your hearing aids. Water is your enemy and can damage the electronics, and many cleaning solvents are too harsh for the hearing aid materials.

WARNING

Avoid using too much pressure to clean your hearing aids. Let the soft bristle brush and cloth do the work without force. When in doubt about cleaning, seek help.

Inspection

It's a good idea to inspect your hearing aid after a cleaning. Look for any signs of wear and tear, including cracks in the body of the hearing aid or tubing. If the hearing aid is a receiver in the canal (see Chapter 9) style, make sure there are no twists or bends in the wire. If the hearing aid uses a dome, check the dome for any tears or stiffness. Replace the dome if it is torn or stiff.

Consult your hearing aid manual or hearing care professional if you notice anything out of the ordinary. A daily once-over can go a long way in preventing bigger problems down the road.

Wax guards

Wax guards are little basket filters that sit in the opening at the end of the hearing aid that goes into the ear canal. They trap wax to prevent it from getting into the electronic components of the hearing aid or into the tube.

Different hearing aid brands have different styles of wax traps. Consult your professional or your hearing aid manual for information on replacing wax traps and purchasing additional wax traps when needed.

TIP

There is no way to predict how regularly someone will need to replace wax guards; each person is different. Using a dryer and brushing daily will certainly help keep wax from building up quickly. Gauging just how full a wax guard is and whether it needs replacement can be difficult. If you turn the hearing aids on and don't hear any sound, a full wax guard is one of your prime suspects.

Avoiding situations that are bad for your hearing aids

Many situations can damage your hearing aids. Water and moisture, excessive heat, and puppies that like to chew anything they can find are hearing aids' arch nemeses. Here are some helpful tips and situations to avoid to keep your hearing aids safe:

>> Remove your hearing aids when you shower, bathe, or swim.

>> Don't store your hearing aids in places they could get wet such as the kitchen or the bathroom.

>> Avoid the steam room and sauna when wearing hearing aids.

>> Take out your hearing aids when you use a hair dryer.

>> Never leave your hearing aids in overly hot places such as the car on a hot, sunny summer day or near a hot stove.

>> Remove your hearing aids when getting any imaging like an MRI.

>> Don't allow hair spray or perfume to come in contact with your hearing aids. Wait for hair care products to dry before putting in your hearing aids.

>> Keep your hearing aids where pets and small children can't get to them. Pets are known to chew on hearing aids!

>> If possible, avoid sleeping with your hearing aids inserted, as they can be crushed or lost. It's best to store your hearing aids in a safe place overnight (especially a dehumidifier or hearing aid dryer).

TIP

It can be easy to make a mistake and forget to remove your hearing aids. This is why creating routines is key. It's a good idea, for example, to create a habit of showering and using a hair dryer before you clean and put in your hearing aids for the day.

Troubleshooting common problems with hearing aids

Life happens, and you will run into problems with your hearing aids. Following are a few common problems and some quick ways to troubleshoot those problems.

REMEMBER

Always consult the hearing aid manual or your hearing care professional if you can't troubleshoot yourself.

There is no sound coming from your hearing aid when you put it in your ear.

>> Check for power. Make sure the battery door is closed or the power switch is on.

>> Check the batteries. If you use disposable batteries, you can purchase a battery tester to see whether they have a charge left. Replace if necessary. If you have rechargeable batteries, the charging station will indicate how much charge the batteries have left.

>> Turn the hearing aid on and off again. We know this is cliché, but it works.

>> Check the volume control if you have one. Make sure it isn't somehow set to mute the hearing aids.

>> Clean your hearing aids and use a magnifying glass to look for wax or debris blocking the microphone, speaker, or tubing.

There is whistling, screeching, buzzing, or feedback.

>> Remove and reinsert the hearing aid into your ear. A loose fit can cause feedback.

>> Clean your hearing aids and look for wax or debris in any openings.

>> Check the hearing aid for any cracks that are allowing sound to leak and cause feedback.

>> Make sure the volume isn't set too high.

TIP

Losing a lot of weight can affect the fit of your domes or earmolds and can cause feedback. In this case, you'll need to either select a different size dome or have a new custom earmold made.

WARNING

Feedback can be caused by wax buildup in your ear. Ask a professional such as an audiologist or ear, nose, and throat physician to look in your ear and remove any wax if needed.

The sound is distorted or cutting in and out.

>> Turn the hearing aid on and off again (we know, we know).

>> Give your hearing aids a good cleaning and make sure there is no moisture in the hearing aid by putting it in the dryer or dehumidifier.

>> Check the battery.

>> If you have a hearing aid with a receiver in the canal (see Chapter 9), check the wire that runs from the hearing aid body to the ear tip that goes in the ear canal for any wear and tear.

>> Check the settings and programs (consult the manual). If you can, try resetting some default settings.

Knowing When It's Time to Upgrade Your Hearing Aid to a New Generation

The most common reason for replacement is that hearing aids are broken or damaged beyond repair. A lot of hearing care professionals will say that hearing aids last around five years, but that may not always be as clear as it sounds. The range can be anywhere from three to ten years, and we don't know how the introduction of OTC hearing aids will impact this range. In general, remember that a good care routine can keep your hearing aids running longer.

The next most common reason for upgrading hearing aids is to get the latest and greatest technology. Hearing aids see annual changes in technology, and most major prescription hearing aid manufacturers release a new line of hearing aids each year. Still, technology evolves incrementally, and you may not always notice a difference when going from one generation of hearing aid technology to the next. Instead, it may be a good idea to wait several generations (three to five years) before exploring an upgrade.

REMEMBER

According to research, higher technology levels do not guarantee better hearing aid benefits. Technology levels in hearing aids are often reflections of lifestyle preferences. Yes, they make hearing aid use more pleasant or easier, but they won't necessarily affect the bottom line when it comes to making you hear better.

A less common reason to upgrade or change hearing aids is when your hearing loss worsens such that you need a more powerful hearing aid. Not all hearing aids can accommodate the needs of more severe hearing losses. This may become a more common reason to upgrade as individuals switch from OTC hearing aids intended for mild to moderate use to prescription hearing aids that can address more severe hearing loss.

TIP

Plan ahead and anticipate your needs a few years down the road. If your hearing loss is on the cusp of needing a more powerful hearing aid, then it may be a good idea to pursue the more powerful device now and allow yourself room to grow over time. Consult a hearing care professional when in doubt.

Chapter **12**

Technology That Boosts Hearing and Hearing Aids

A theme throughout this book is that hearing loss is complex. A lot of factors can affect your hearing. Likewise, there are multiple ways to address hearing loss. Our goal with this book is to give you a tool kit with a wide array of options to meet your needs. Other chapters cover solutions such as communication tips, environmental modifications, and hearing aids.

In this chapter, we add to your hearing care toolkit with what professionals call hearing assistive technology. Some of these options stand alone, such as captioning, smart home devices, and personal sound amplification products. Others pair directly with your hearing aids for a better experience.

Captioning Your Life

You're probably familiar with captioning: the text displayed on a screen from a live or recorded program. Captions can provide speech as well as indications of who is speaking during voiceover narration, background music, or sound effects. Captions can replace or augment spoken speech by helping to fill in the gaps of difficult-to-hear words and phrases.

Using captions on TV

Probably the most well-known captioning is provided on televisions. Universally, TVs provide the option to turn on captions. Prerecorded programs usually are free of errors in the captions, but in live captioning, you'll often spot spelling errors, botched names, and the mixing up of words that sound similar. The U.S. Federal Communications Commission has rules ensuring television distributors such as cable and broadcast television companies provide captions that meet a certain quality of accuracy without too much time lag between spoken speech and the caption text.

Adults with even mild hearing loss and hearing aid users find captioning helpful to make sense of difficult to make our words. In fact, many people without hearing loss use captioning when watching TV because it makes it easier to follow along regardless of whether you have hearing loss or not. Both Frank and Nick are "captions always on" people when watching TVs and movies.

Obtaining and using captioned phones (They're free!)

Captioned telephones have large built-in screens to display the text of what the other person on the call is saying in real time. During the call, a captioned telephone service generates the text using a combination of speech recognition technology and specially trained captioners. Yes, someone is listening in on your calls! (But no need to fret. In the United States, this is a federally regulated public service and all captioners are required to sign confidentiality agreements that are strictly enforced.) Thanks to a federally funded program, adults with hearing loss can obtain a free captioned telephone. All you need is a completed application and a signed certification from a qualified professional, either an audiologist or physician, verifying your hearing loss. Some of the common caption phone companies are CapTel, CaptionCall, ClearCaptions, Hamilton CapTel, and Spring CapTel.

Captioning services are also available for use on your smartphone. To use captioned services, you can download apps in the Apple or Android app store such as CaptionCall App or InnoCaption App. You will then make and receive calls through these apps, which will then automatically connect you with a trained captioner. Alternatively, smartphones can use automated captioning that can provide captions during phone calls. These are turned on via the accessibility or volume settings on your smartphone. Google smartphones, for example, let you turn their captioning service (LiveCaption) on right under the volume adjustment. However, be warned that these automatic algorithms may make mistakes that a trained live captioner would avoid.

TIP

Many different companies offer free captioning services for phone calls. The Hearing Loss Association of America maintains a listing of the various companies to which you can apply: www.hearingloss.org/hearing-help/technology/phones-mobile-devices/.

Captioning in video conference calls

Captioning during video conference calls can provide another layer of information to help you understand spoken speech.

Many video conference call platforms such as Cisco Webex, Google Meet, Microsoft Teams, Skype, and Zoom have their own automated live caption services. There are also third-party automated captioning providers such as OtterAI. The services use automated voice recognition technology and are not regulated by any government agency. Again, they're not perfect; you'll likely spot many errors in the text. But the technology is still helpful and constantly improving.

TIP

For some video conferencing platforms, only the host (the person who schedules the call or someone that person assigns) can turn on the captions. If you're the host, always remember to turn on captions. If you're a guest and captioning isn't on, advocate for yourself (and others!) and ask the host to turn on captioning.

CART for live sessions

If you're planning or attending a live or remote meeting and want to provide captioning, consider communication access real-time translation (CART) services. CART is the name for the system that specially trained writers or stenographers use to convert speech to text in real time. The writers use a special phonetic keyboard that uses speech sounds instead of letters to write words. By focusing on the sounds instead of letters, the writers can produce rapid and highly accurate captions.

CART services are the gold standard for providing real-time captioning during live events with speakers, either online or in-person, such as at a conference.

TIP

You can search online for CART service providers near you. Just a tip: When searching the web, write out "communication access real-time translation" in a search engine or risk getting back a lot of golf cart rental websites. Once you've hired a CART service, here are some tips to prepare for the event:

>> Provide the CART writers with any material (such as slides and handouts) to help them familiarize themselves with the topic and prepare ahead of time.

>> Make sure the screen for the text is large and visible to everyone.

>> Consider doubling up CART captions with direct audio streaming technology such as a hearing loop to provide multiple options for the audience. Most people do best with simultaneous visual and audio options.

Outfitting Your Home with Hearing-Friendly Tech

We spend a lot of time in our home, so it makes sense for us to design it to meet our own hearing needs and preferences. Since the early days of hearing technology, there has been home-based assistive technology. Over time, that technology has improved. Today, hearing assistive technology has been integrated into the modern "smart home" options that use internet connections to control many home functions (such as thermostats, doorbells, and lighting) through smartphone apps. Following are some options for hearing assistive technology in the home:

>> Doorbells can use blinking lights or connect to your smartphone to alert you to someone at the door.

>> Alarm clocks can add extra loud alarms, vibrations, or bright lights.

>> Captioned telephones provide for real-time text display of your phone conversations. Check out the earlier section "Obtaining and using captioned phones (They're free!)."

>> TV sound boxes and wireless headsets allow you to get a louder and more direct signal.

>> Smoke and carbon monoxide detectors come in models that have extra-loud alarms and flashing lights to alert you of any smoke or toxins.

>> Smart light systems can be integrated with other products to blink or change color to alert you to something. For example, smart lights could be set to blink when the oven is preheated, turn blue and blink to alert you to an incoming phone call, or turn red in the case of a fire.

>> Handheld personal sound amplifiers placed around the house can serve as a way to magnify sound when you or a guest need a boost. Even if you have hearing aids, it's useful to have handheld amplifiers as a backup.

TIP

Good lighting can go a long way in improving conversation as it helps to be able to see people's faces when they are speaking.

Talking about Integration Technology

Bluetooth technology and the wide array of smartphone apps make customizing strategies to aid in improving day-to-day functions with hearing loss a whole lot easier.

Working with Bluetooth and hearing aids

Bluetooth is amazing wireless connection technology. It is a short-range wireless connection platform that allows data transfer or connections between two or more electronic devices over ultra-high frequency radio waves that don't interfere with other signals. Thousands of companies across the globe, including hearing aid manufacturers, have agreed on Bluetooth as the standard in wireless connection and have teamed up to form a special interest group that manages the technology, fosters Bluetooth tech advances, and maintains high security standards.

Bluetooth allows hearing aids to directly connect to other devices, including smartphones and tablets, to stream clear audio such as music or phone calls. Many hearing aid companies now offer smartphone apps that connect to hearing aids via Bluetooth and allow the user to control hearing aid settings such as volume and programs or check on the hearing aid battery life.

TIP

Most hearing aids connect to smartphones by making sure Bluetooth is activated on the smartphone and then turning the hearing aid off and back on. This prompts the two devices to pair. After the first connection, the devices will remember one another and automatically pair. Consult your hearing aid user manual, contact a tech savvy friend, or ask your hearing care professional when in doubt.

WARNING

Some hearing aids require a streamer (see the section "Streaming all your devices," later in this chapter) to connect to other devices via Bluetooth. This is usually worn around the neck or kept in a pocket. But this is becoming increasingly rare as modern technology allows for a direct connection. Check product labels or speak with a hearing professional for how hearing aids connect to Bluetooth if you want to avoid using an extra device.

Navigating smartphone apps

You can find many, many smartphone apps for hearing loss — some free, some not — and it can be difficult to distinguish the good from the not-so-good. There are two main categories specific to enhancing your hearing:

>> Apps to amplify sounds in your environment just like a handheld amplifier

>> Apps to customize sound you listen to through your smartphone, such as when you take calls or stream music, so that it is tailored to your hearing

But how do you know whether an app is going to be reliable? Here are some tips:

>> Look for apps that are popular and have lots of downloads.

>> Read reviews and comments by users.

>> Download apps only from official app stores.

>> Look at apps that have a history of regularly updating.

>> Pay attention to permissions the app asks for on your phone; predatory apps may ask for permission to access unnecessary information (like an app to amplify sound requesting access to your photos or contacts).

Checking Out Hearing Aid Accessories

Hearing aid accessories can be the difference between doing okay and thriving with hearing aids. Many companies offer a lineup of complementary accessories that can boost your experience with hearing aids and improve listening in certain situations. Every company has a different specific name for these products, but there are four common types: a remote control, a remote microphone, a TV connector, and a streamer.

Using a remote control

A remote control acts as a handheld operations center for your hearing aids. It allows you to discretely control your hearing aids without needing to locate and press any buttons on the hearing aids themselves. This can be especially useful for adults with stiff, numb, or arthritic fingers. With a remote control you can:

>> Adjust the volume or mute the hearing aids.

>> Change the programs to match the situation you're in.

>> Manage connections to other streaming devices.

Trying out a remote microphone

A remote microphone is a stand-alone or portable microphone that transmits a direct signal to hearing aids from a distance. Remote microphones excel in helping with hearing in difficult listening environments from noise or overcoming distance issues. Hearing aids can mute or dampen any other sounds around you while focusing only on the remote microphone to substantially improve clarity.

Remote microphones are one of our favorite accessories and something we recommend to almost every hearing aid user who has trouble with hearing aids in noisy situations. We compare the remote microphone for those with extra trouble with speech in noise to using snow tires for driving in cold weather areas: It's a must-have accessory!

There are two main styles of remote microphone: one-on-one remote mic and group setting remote mic.

One-on-one remote mic

The most common style is a portable personal microphone for focused conversation when you're only interested in hearing one specific person speak at a time. The person speaking can hold it, wear it around their neck, or clip it to their shirt or jacket lapel. The sound from the microphone is channeled directly into your hearing aid. Let's go through some examples of when the remote microphone comes in handy:

>> If you are at a noisy restaurant for dinner, you can have the person you're dining with wear the remote microphone so that you receive a more direct signal of their voice with less background noise.

>> In some social settings with lots of noise, like a large gathering or at a bar, we tend to move from conversation to conversation. You can bring the one-on-one remote microphone and either hold it yourself near the person (see Figure 12-1) or ask the person you're speaking with to hold to it for a boosted signal.

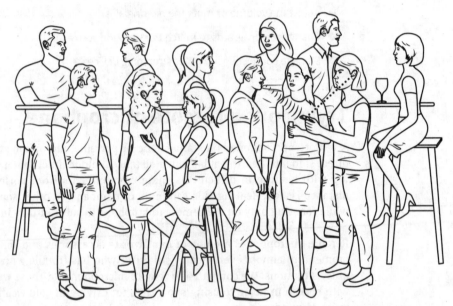

FIGURE 12-1:
The portable
remote
microphone
being held while
at a party.

Source: John Wiley & Sons, Inc.

>> Lectures can be difficult if you're forced to sit far away from the speaker. Even if the venue has a sound system, it can still be difficult to understand the speaker depending on the acoustics as well as the quality and placement of the speakers. You can either place the remote microphone on the podium or request the speaker wear it to give you a direct signal (see Figure 12-2). The range on remote microphones varies from roughly 30 to 90 feet depending on the manufacturer.

TIP

If you're in a small group setting with the one-on-one remote mic, like a noisy restaurant with a group of three, you can try placing the microphone on the table between your dining companions or ask them to pass it back and forth as needed. It's an extra step but will make for a smoother and more enjoyable conversation for everyone.

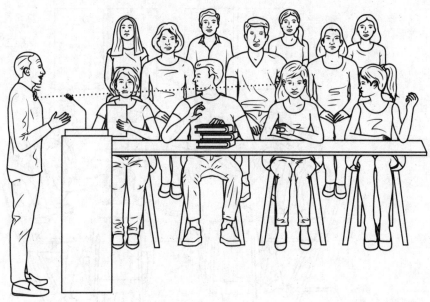

Source: John Wiley & Sons, Inc.

FIGURE 12-2:
The one-on-one remote microphone in action during a lecture.

Group setting remote mic

A newer version of the remote microphone is a table remote microphone that is specially designed for group conversations. This product sits on a table and uses a combination of advanced signal processing and special microphones called *beamformers* to identify and focus on anyone speaking at the table and transmit that signal directly to your hearing aids.

The table remote microphone is a great option when in a restaurant or at home with multiple people or for use at work meetings around a conference table (see Figure 12-3). At the publication of this book, this is a newer product and is only available through a few hearing aid manufacturers, but the initial popularity among patients suggests it's going to quickly become a widely offered product.

Connecting to the TV

The TV connector serves a very specific role of transmitting the audio signal from any home audio device, namely TVs and stereos, directly to your hearing aids (see Figure 12-4). Simply plug the TV connector into the audio port on your TV or stereo to connect to your hearing aids. This can make listening to TV much more enjoyable with a direct and sometimes clearer signal compared to using your hearing aids alone. Many companies now offer the capability for the TV connector to stream to multiple sets of hearing aids if you are watching TV with a friend or family member!

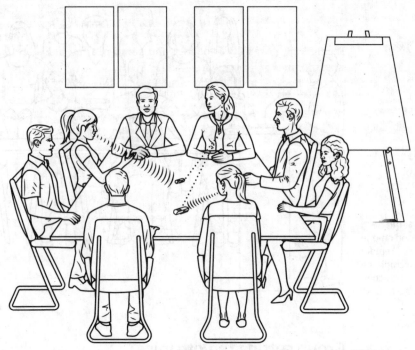

FIGURE 12-3:
The table remote
microphone
during a meeting.

Source: John Wiley & Sons, Inc.

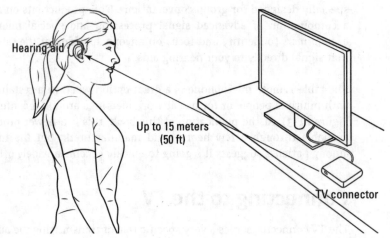

Hearing aid

Up to 15 meters
(50 ft)

TV connector

FIGURE 12-4:
The TV connector
plugs into the TV
and sends a
direct signal to
your hearing aids.

Source: John Wiley & Sons, Inc.

Streaming all your devices

Technology is rapidly evolving, and some hearing aids can directly connect to smartphones and other accessories mentioned in this section. However, some hearing aids will require a streamer (see Figure 12-5) to act as an intermediary transmitter to allow hearing aids to connect to other products. The streamer is usually worn around a hearing aid user's neck or kept in their pocket. For some hearing aid manufacturers, the streamer and remote control are combined into a single product to make your life easier. Make sure you do a little research first to find out if your hearing aids require a streamer to connect to accessories and your smartphone.

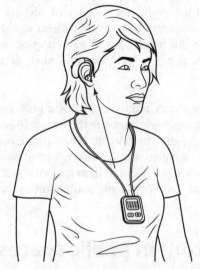

Source: John Wiley & Sons, Inc.

FIGURE 12-5:
The streamer is worn around the wearer's neck.

WARNING

When purchasing hearing aid accessories, make sure they are compatible with your hearing aids. At the time of this book, most hearing aids are only compatible with accessories made by the same manufacturer. Even within a single manufacturer, new generation technology does not always work with older technology. You can always ask your hearing care professional to help you navigate the accessories market.

The Mighty Telecoil: Getting a Direct Connection to Sound Signals

The telecoil is an option in hearing aids that allows for a direct connection to sound with telephones and in some public places. It is one of the oldest hearing aid features still in regular use and has been a popular option since it was first added as a feature in hearing aids in the 1970s. We highly recommend getting hearing aids that have telecoils.

The name telecoil refers to an actual part in the hearing aid. During the manufacturing process, a small, coiled (hence the name) copper wire is placed inside the hearing aid. The coil picks up on electromagnetic signals generated from compatible communication equipment to transmit a direct signal to your hearing aids. The two main uses for the telecoil are in gathering places with specially installed systems called hearing loops (see the next section) and with telephones.

Many hearing aids can detect a telecoil-compatible signal and automatically switch into telecoil mode while some will require the wearer to either press a button or use a remote control to use the telecoil. When the telecoil is active, the hearing aid will dampen other ambient sounds. This is a great way to get a focused auditory signal because it means the signal of interest (what you want to hear) is boosted while the background noise (what you don't want to hear) is untouched or dampened.

Looping in telecoils in public spaces

Some public spaces, such as places of worship, auditoriums or large classrooms, theaters, museums, healthcare offices, airports, or train and subway stations, have installed hearing loop systems. These locations will have signs to indicate telecoil compatibility (see Figure 12-7). If you are wearing a hearing aid with a telecoil in a looped area, your hearing aid will either automatically detect the signal and switch to telecoil mode, or you will need to press a button to activate telecoil mode. This will allow for direct streaming of audio signals to your hearing aids.

TIP

Look for the universal hearing loop sign (see Figure 12-6) when out and about or check out hearingloop.org to learn more about loops and to search for looped spaces near you. Loops are more common in Europe than the United States, but they are increasing in popularity in the United States.

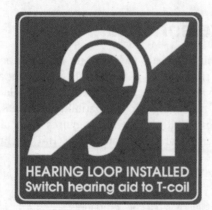

FIGURE 12-6: A sign with the universal symbol indicating an area is telecoil compatable.

Figure 12-7 shows a hearing loop system in an auditorium or large classroom in action. The pre-installed hearing loop runs the perimeter of the classroom. The lecturer's words are picked up by a pre-installed microphone and transmitted directly to your hearing aids via the hearing loss amplifier. Alternatively, hearing loops can be used to transmit auditory signals that are prerecorded like information about train or airplane departure times in public transportation settings.

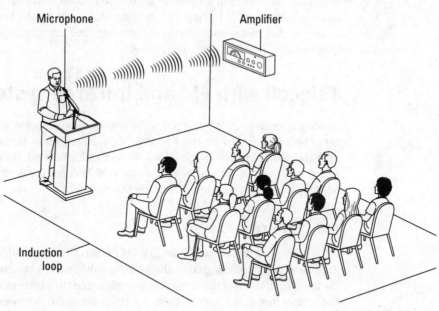

Microphone

Amplifier

FIGURE 12-7: Induction loop system in a large classroom.

Induction loop

Source: John Wiley & Sons, Inc.

Telecoils and telephones

At the advent of the telecoil, phones — which were landlines at the time — all emitted a magnetic signal that worked with telecoils. That's not a given today. If you're purchasing a phone and want to know whether it has telecoil capabilities, you'll need to check the packaging for compatibility. In 1988, U.S. Congress passed the Hearing Aid Compatibility Act, which requires many phones and other communication devices to use hearing aid compatible (HAC) technology.

There are two HAC ratings: T and M:

>> The T rating means the device is telecoil compatible.

>> The M rating means the device is compatible with hearing aids without using the telecoil.

Both ratings also include a scale from 1 to 4 after the M or T with 4 representing the "best" or "highest" rating of compatibility. Thus, a T4 rating indicates the best compatibility with a hearing aid telecoil.

WARNING

If you are interested in a hearing aid with a telecoil, ask your hearing care professional, or if you're buying OTC hearing aids, look for the feature on the label. Be aware that some manufacturers have removed the telecoil to save space and make smaller hearing aids. Always check first.

Telecoil with FM and infrared systems

Instead of hearing loop systems, some gathering spaces use frequency modulation (FM) or infrared systems to provide a direct audio signal for people with hearing loss. Unlike the hearing loop system with a telecoil, these systems require extra equipment to connect with hearing aids. Many of those options require your hearing aids to have a telecoil for direct audio streaming.

FM systems

FM systems use radio waves (just like FM radio) to transmit audio signals that can provide a direct audio signal in the hearing aids. The FM system works by having the speaker of interest use a microphone connected to a transmitter that sends out the audio signal via radio waves to the immediate surrounding area within approximately 30 to 90 feet.

Hearing aids have to be outfitted with a special FM receiver to pick up the audio signal. There are two main options to connect with hearing aids:

>> A small FM receiver can be attached to the bottom of behind-the-ear style (see Chapter 9) hearing aids. It just slightly extends the length of the hearing aid.

>> A loop can be worn around the hearing aid wearer's neck and transmit the signal to the hearing aid via the telecoil. But this requires that the hearing aids have a telecoil.

Infrared systems

Infrared systems look a lot like FM systems except they transmit sound via light signals (yes, you read that right). The system uses a microphone to pick up a speaker's voice, which is sent to a transmitter that converts the sound signal to light energy and sends it out into the immediate surroundings. Special infrared receivers pick up the signal and turn the light energy back into sound. This seems like a lot of coding and decoding, but the advantage is that the light signals aren't subject to interference from other audio signals like radio wave transmissions, which can happen with FM systems.

Just like with FM systems, hearing aids require extra equipment to connect to infrared systems. This usually takes the form of a neck loop that then sends the signal to the telecoil.

Pros and cons of each system

Overall, there are advantages and disadvantages to FM systems and infrared systems. Both are a practical option for people without telecoils in their hearing aids. And they are easier and less costly to install compared to the hearing loop. FM systems are even portable! In fact, FM systems are a favorite in primary and secondary school systems because of their portability and affordability. However, both systems require hearing aid users to wear an extra piece of equipment for direct audio streaming. For those who don't have a telecoil in their hearing aids or don't have hearing aids at all but are still interested in a boost, venues that offer FM systems and infrared systems can offer large headsets that connect directly to the signal. These look like the headsets you might receive on guided tours in a museum.

Has Bluetooth replaced telecoils? (No!)

As Bluetooth has become more popular, some have suggested that telecoils are now outdated since they're both forms of wireless connection technology for a direct audio signal in hearing aids. This could not be further from the truth!

Bluetooth is great and can offer superior sound quality, but it does not yet offer the same range as telecoils to offer, doesn't cover large public spaces, and can quickly drain the battery of any device using it for a connection, including hearing aids. Each has its own advantages and disadvantages. Currently, Bluetooth and telecoils both have a place in hearing aid technology.

Sounding Out Personal Amplifiers

You may have seen advertisements about devices called personal sound amplification products (PSAPs). PSAPs make sound louder, with the term "amplify" right there in the name. Some even look just like hearing aids. It can be hard to distinguish between a PSAP and a hearing aid. In this section, we walk you through the differences to help you decide whether they are right for you.

Demystifying PSAPs versus hearing aids

So, if PSAPs can amplify sound and look just like hearing aids, then what makes them different? The key difference between PSAPs and hearing aids boils down to regulation and intended use.

Both prescription and OTC hearing aids are regulated and approved by the U.S. Food and Drug Administration (FDA) as devices intended to treat and address hearing loss. This means that hearing aids have to meet minimum standards set by the FDA so they can legally advertise as being for people with hearing loss.

PSAPs are unregulated devices with no specific criteria, which means PSAPs *cannot* claim to treat or compensate for hearing loss. Instead, PSAPs are intended to make sound louder and help with listening in certain situations for people with normal hearing.

PSAPs are commonly advertised to help in the following situations: watching birds, hunting, listening to speakers from a distance, or talking to someone in a tough listening environment like a hospital. Wait, don't these sound familiar? Many of these situations are the same things we've talked about using hearing aids for throughout this entire book.

Believe us, we're just as confused as you.

The reality is that people with normal hearing and with hearing loss participate in the same activities, so PSAPs can advertise to amplify sound in those settings. The difference is nuanced in that these advertisements are very situationally specific and not focused on treating hearing loss across all aspects of someone's life.

The reality of using PSAPs

Let's get this out of the way: If you were to put either Frank or Nick's name into an internet search engine, you're going to see them talking about using PSAPs for hearing loss. This is because we believe that any help is better than no help.

On paper, hearing aids are for hearing loss and PSAPs are not. But the reality is much more nuanced, and PSAPs are regularly used to address hearing loss, especially in specific situations. In fact, the most famous PSAP might be the handheld amplifier, often referred to as Pocketalker, that is commonly seen in health care settings and regularly recommended for helping patients with hearing loss communicate with their doctors.

Products are increasingly blurring the line between being just situational amplifiers versus something that could also help with hearing loss across multiple settings. For example, researchers at the National Acoustic Laboratories in Australia have shown that Apple AirPods Pro are capable of customizing sound with enough amplification and manipulation that they could feasibly be used for adults with mild to moderate hearing loss. Our own team at Johns Hopkins University has shown that some PSAPs are capable of comparable results to hearing aids in improving hearing for adults with mild to moderate hearing loss.

REMEMBER

The bottom line is that a PSAP could be a good option if you have mild to moderate hearing loss, especially if you're looking for something that is situational specific. PSAPs are not an option for adults with more severe hearing loss. And pursuing PSAPs will be a gamble to some extent because they are unregulated and not required to meet any standards.

Navigating the unregulated amplifier marketplace

PSAPs can be sold directly to a consumer without needing to go through a professional. Cost varies drastically but a rough range is between $30 and $400 per device.

WARNING

More reality for you: Some high-quality PSAPs are capable of helping with hearing loss but the majority of the PSAP market is, well, just plain crummy. Most PSAPs are not going to help with hearing loss and several of the really bad PSAPs produce sound that is so distorted it can make hearing with hearing loss more difficult.

That's the nature of a completely unregulated market — there may be some good products but there will be plenty of bad products. We recommend you proceed with some caution. It can be really hard to navigate the PSAP market and it will require some research to find a good product. Some things to look for:

>> Products that have overwhelmingly positive reviews on internet sales websites

>> A company that offers warranties

>> A company that has a clearly written manual and offers some information about the technical specifications of the product

>> Positive commentary from third-party organizations that test products, like Consumer Reports or Wirecutter

Will OTC hearing aids replace PSAPs?

Some wonder whether the new OTC hearing aids, available without seeing a professional, will make PSAPs go the way of the dodo. No, PSAPs aren't going anywhere. Consumer electronic companies will continue to make various amplification devices, and some will be pretty amazing. While we don't expect that the OTC hearing aid category will replace PSAPs altogether, it could affect the layout of the PSAP marketplace.

The new OTC hearing aid category will be regulated by the FDA with a set of minimum standards to ensure they are appropriate for treating mild to moderate hearing loss in adults. This means OTC hearing aids will offer a level of reassurance that the PSAP market does not have. For example, if you were shopping for a hearing device and saw a PSAP and an OTC hearing aid next to one another, you would see the label that the OTC hearing aid is "Food and Drug Administration approved" and language around being for "mild to moderate hearing loss." Those are comforting statements if you're looking for the best product to address hearing loss.

Some PSAP companies with quality products that can meet the minimum criteria may choose to pursue OTC hearing aid status just to make sure their products have those labels.

Chapter **13**

Medical and Surgical Treatment of Hearing Loss

Frankly, not many people will need to use medication and surgical options for treating the types of hearing loss we cover in this chapter. These situations aren't that common relative to the number of people (almost everyone!) who will develop hearing loss over time, but they're important to know about.

For these options, you'll need to consult an otolaryngologist (also known as an ear, nose, and throat, or ENT, doctor) rather than an audiologist or hearing instrument specialist.

In this chapter, we tell you about medications for certain conditions and surgical devices to help with hearing.

Looking into Medications That Treat Hearing Loss

If you're having trouble with your hearing, there are only a few instances where medications might help, which we cover in this section. For most hearing loss related to aging, we're sorry to say, there's definitely no miracle drug on the horizon in the next five to ten years (see the nearby sidebar "A fountain of youth for the ear?").

Using steroids for sudden hearing loss

Steroids are the rare exception of a medication that may be used for sensorineural hearing loss. This type of drug may be indicated in instances when someone experiences a sudden sensorineural hearing loss (see Chapter 3). In these cases, the sudden sensorineural hearing loss may be related to an infection of the inner ear with a virus or in rarer cases an autoimmune disease.

Taking steroids in these situations may help reduce inflammation and allow the cochlea and related hearing function to recover. The key word to note in the last sentence, though, is "may."

The scientific evidence for how well steroids work in these situations is limited. Studies are really hard to do because these types of sudden hearing loss are rare.

Regardless, though, the vast majority of ENTs (Frank included) still generally recommend a course of steroids for patients who experience a sudden loss of hearing that is confirmed on an audiogram.

Steroids are generally administered in pill form that you take by mouth for 10 to 14 days. Alternatively, your ENT can inject the steroid directly through a microscopic hole in your eardrum, where it then gets absorbed into the inner ear. This is a routine procedure that is done in the ENT office that is not much different (and no more painful!) than getting earwax cleaned out of your ear.

To have the best chance of success, these steroid treatments must be given as soon as possible — ideally within three days — after the onset of hearing loss.

REMEMBER

If you ever feel that your hearing in one ear (it almost never happens in both ears at the same time) suddenly is gone, you should be seen within ideally three and no more than five days by an ENT to get your hearing evaluated and to start on possible steroid therapy. This is one of the few ENT emergencies where it's critical to be seen promptly. The diagnosis of a sudden sensorineural hearing loss is made based on a diagnostic audiogram conducted by an audiologist followed by an examination with an ENT.

Taking medications for problems with the external or middle ear

Infections of the external or middle ear can lead to a temporary conductive hearing loss — that is, when sounds can't effectively travel through the eardrum and middle ear bones to the inner ear. Medications can be used in these situations to help treat the infection and resolve the conductive hearing loss.

Infections of the middle ear happen when fluid collects in the middle ear space (this space is normally filled with air), and this process often results from swelling around the Eustachian tube opening related to a cold or allergies (see Chapter 3). An infection of the external ear canal can also sometimes lead to a temporary conductive hearing loss if the ear canal and ear drum become sufficiently swollen to prevent sound from getting through.

A FOUNTAIN OF YOUTH FOR THE EAR?

Ahh . . . if only we could all just take a drug that would miraculously restore our hearing back to our teenage years.

Well, we're not quite there yet, but such drugs are undergoing early testing and development now. Many pharmaceutical company startups are working on drugs that could potentially turn on the inner ear's ability to regenerate the cells needed for hearing and potentially reverse hearing loss. That said, as of 2022, nothing is remotely on the horizon within the next five years for widespread use, and some skeptical clinicians and scientists may say these types of restorative therapies *always* seem to be five to ten years away.

The reason for this skepticism is that as with any part of the body (or any machine in fact), it's always harder to undo damage (or restore function) once the damage has been done. The ear is likely no different, and in particular, hearing loss that develops over time directly reflects damage to the ear that has accumulated over many years, making it much harder to reverse.

The most likely future scenario is that drugs eventually become available to help restore hearing, but they may be indicated for only very specific types of hearing loss. For example, drugs being developed now may help only very specific types of rare genetic hearing loss in children or help prevent hearing loss for those who take a chemotherapy drug for cancer that could damage the inner ear.

If you notice pain, swelling of the ear canal, or drainage coming from the affected ear, you may have an external or middle ear infection. These symptoms may happen after water exposure to the ear (which can lead to an external ear infection) or while having allergies or a cold (which can affect the Eustachian tube).

In the case of external or middle ear infection, your primary care doctor or an ENT may prescribe oral antibiotics or some type of antibiotic ear drops to fight the infection. In the case of swelling around the Eustachian tube, your doctor may have you try a nasal steroid spray or nasal saline rinse to try to decrease any inflammation or swelling in your nose that may be contributing to blockage around the Eustachian tube opening.

Checking Out Different Surgeries for Hearing Loss

Similar to medications for hearing loss, existing surgeries for hearing loss can be either for conditions involving the external or middle ear that prevent sounds from getting through (conductive hearing loss) or for inner ear issues (sensorineural hearing loss, where the cochlea is not converting the sounds clearly to send to the brain).

Surgeries for conductive hearing loss

Problems with the external and middle ear that can lead to a conductive hearing loss and possibly be helped by surgery include the following:

>> **Stiffening of the ear bones:** The three ear bones of the middle ear can stiffen in place, preventing sound from getting through. This most commonly results from frequent middle ear infections, or a process called otosclerosis that can run in families and leads to the stapes ear bone becoming fixated in place.

>> **Chronic fluid in the middle ear (also called a *middle ear effusion*):** Most collections of fluid in the middle ear are temporary and last only a few weeks once the swelling around the Eustachian tube, from a cold or nasal allergies, resolves and the fluid can drain out. If the fluid persists for more than 2 to 3 months, a minor surgical procedure may be considered to drain the fluid by making a small incision in the eardrum.

>> **Eardrum perforation:** A hole in the eardrum can often result from previous infections or trauma to the ear canal (most commonly from a cotton swab or other object placed in the ear canal that then goes too deep).

>> **Cholesteatoma:** If an eardrum perforation is present along with persistent ear infections, skin from outside the eardrum can grow into the middle ear and slowly erode away the ear bones and other structures.

Based on audiological testing, physical examination of your ear, and possibly a CT scan of your ear, an ENT surgeon may recommend surgery to repair these problems of the external and middle ear depending on the severity of the condition and symptoms you may be experiencing.

Surgery for sensorineural hearing loss

Sensorineural hearing losses can generally not be treated with surgery with the notable exception of someone who has severe sensorineural hearing loss (see Chapter 7), which generally corresponds to a hearing number (pure-tone average) in the 60s or higher, and who is not finding sufficient benefit from using hearing aids. The main surgical option for treating such types of severe sensorineural hearing loss is cochlear implantation.

A cochlear implant (CI) is the most widely used neuroprosthetic device (*neuro*, relating to the nervous system; *prosthetic*, meaning an engineered device that takes the place of a body part — in this case, the cochlea) ever created and has been around since the late 1980s. To date, well more than 200,000 Americans have received a cochlear implant.

What is a cochlear implant and how does it work?

A CI is a surgically implanted device that converts sound into an electrical signal. The device takes over the usual role of the cochlea in converting sound into a neural (electrical) signal that goes to the brain.

A CI comprises both an internal implant and an external component. The internal implant consists of an electrode array, receiver, and internal magnet that is placed under the skin during a routine outpatient surgery. The external component consists of the speech processor and transmitter coil that also contains a magnet, which allows the transmitter to "stick" to the side of the head opposite the internal magnet that is under the skin. See Figure 13-1.

Sound is picked up by the external speech processor, where it's converted to an electrical code. This code is then transmitted wirelessly through the transmitter coil to the internal receiver and relayed via the electrode array to the hearing nerve that goes to the brain.

This process results in sound being sent straight to the brain and can allow someone who could barely hear to suddenly have access to sound and language again!

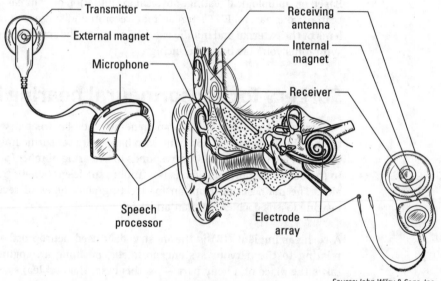

FIGURE 13-1: A cochlear implant.

Source: John Wiley & Sons, Inc.

Who is a candidate for a cochlear implant?

A CI is typically considered for individuals with a severe sensorineural hearing loss (hearing number in the 60s or greater; see Chapter 7) who can no longer obtain adequate benefit from a conventional hearing aid. This happens when there's been enough damage to the cochlea that the signals being sent from the cochlea to the brain (even with the help of a good hearing aid) remain difficult to understand under many common daily situations.

Individuals who could potentially benefit from a cochlear implant may still find they can get by with a hearing aid under ideal circumstances (such as speaking face-to-face with a familiar speaker in a completely quiet room), but communication quickly breaks down in other circumstances.

Many people continue to struggle with hearing aids for years before considering a CI, thinking that their hearing is still "too good" to get a CI. As a result, researchers estimate that only about 5 to 10 percent of adults who could qualify for a CI end up getting one.

REMEMBER

If you've ever been told that you have a severe hearing loss (with a hearing number in the 60s or worse) and you feel that you're struggling to hear and communicate with hearing aids, we highly recommend that you get evaluated to see if you may be a good candidate for a cochlear implant.

In the past, CIs were typically considered only when the hearing in both ears was poor, but increasingly over the past few years, people with single-sided deafness (for example, one ear still has normal hearing, but the other ear has severe hearing loss) are also getting CIs with good success. Researchers are increasingly understanding the importance of hearing with both ears in order to effectively hear and communicate, particularly in challenging listening conditions (see Chapter 2).

What to expect with a cochlear implant

CIs are miraculous technology, but it's important to be realistic about what a CI can and can't do. A CI will *not* restore your hearing to what it was like when you were a teenager in high school. A CI *will* give you far more access to sound than a hearing aid and allow you to communicate and to engage with the world a whole lot easier.

The surgery to implant the device is a routine outpatient surgery conducted by an ENT (typically one who specializes in otology or neurotology). First, surgery is performed to place the internal implant. Next, a few weeks later (after the surgical site heals), the implant is turned on during an appointment with the cochlear implant audiologist. It then takes a person about 6 to 12 months to get used to hearing with the implant and achieve maximal benefit in hearing.

An analogy for a CI is to think about someone who may have had their lower leg amputated because of an injury. The person may be able to get around okay on crutches, but a far better solution in many cases is to be fitted for a prosthetic leg. When the prosthetic leg is first fitted, the person can't yet walk on it, but with physical therapy and training, the person is generally able to walk well again, and some individuals may even go on to engage in sports and compete in races. The prosthetic leg is certainly not the same as having their native leg, but it's a lot better than crutches!

The same principles apply for a CI. When the CI is first turned on, the sounds the brain hears from the implant may sound strange, and it takes a person about 6 to 12 months working with their CI audiologist to get used to these sounds. Similar to a prosthetic leg, the CI won't be as good as having your native hearing back, but it's often far better than a hearing aid in allowing a person to communicate and engage with the world.

How to get evaluated for a CI

Academic centers and specialized private ENT practices with expertise in otology or neurotology often perform CIs. If you have a severe hearing loss with a hearing number score around 60 or worse (see Chapter 7) or you feel that you're often struggling to communicate even with hearing aids, it's worth getting formally evaluated at a CI center to see whether you're a candidate. At this appointment, a CI audiologist will conduct various hearing and speech tests to see if you qualify for a cochlear implant. CIs are fortunately routinely covered in the United States by Medicare and private insurance plans.

Additional information about CIs, the evaluation process, and how to identify a local cochlear implant clinic is available at the American Cochlear Implant Alliance's website at www.acialliance.org.

Other surgically implantable hearing devices

Cochlear implants are far and away one of the most common implantable hearing devices, but there are a variety of other implantable hearing devices as well. While we don't exhaustively go over all these devices here, the general description that applies to most of them is that they are *osseointegrated* — that is, surgically implanted into the bone — hearing devices.

How these devices work

These devices have a small implant component typically about the size of a thumbtack that is surgically implanted (*osseointegrated*) into the bone behind the ear. An external sound processor is attached to this implant (see Figure 13-2). This processor picks up external sounds and sends them to the implant as vibrations, which are then transmitted directly to the bone of the skull and the cochlea. Unlike a cochlear implant, an osseointegrated hearing device depends on a functioning cochlea to still be able to convert the vibrations into a neural signal.

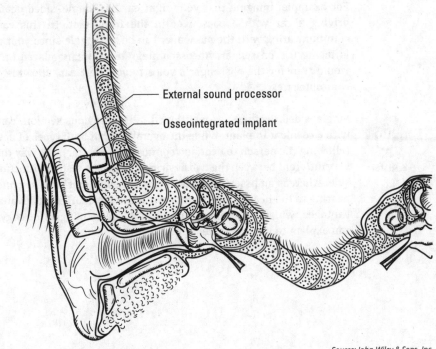

External sound processor

Osseointegrated implant

FIGURE 13-2:
An osseointegrated implant.

Source: John Wiley & Sons, Inc.

Depending on the manufacturer and type of osseointegrated implant, the implant can be inserted directly through the skin into the bone behind the ear in a simple outpatient surgery. There are also newer types of osseointegrated implants where the entire implant lies under the skin and the external processor is attached via a magnet (so nothing is visible on the skin surface when the processor is taken off).

Who these hearing devices are for

These types of implantable hearing devices are often used in people who have a conductive hearing loss from a damaged eardrum, have ear bones that can't be surgically fixed, or for different reasons can't benefit from using a conventional hearing aid. In these cases, an osseointegrated implant can send amplified sound straight to the cochlea.

You may also be a candidate for one of these devices if you have one non-hearing ear (also termed single-sided deafness). In these cases, the device is surgically implanted on the side with the non-hearing ear, so sounds are transmitted to the hearing ear.

For example, imagine that your right ear has single-sided deafness and you're driving a car with a passenger in the front seat. In this case, hearing and communicating with the passenger can be a struggle since your non-hearing ear is facing the passenger. An osseointegrated implant placed on your right side would transfer the passenger's voice to your left ear, allowing you to hear and communicate.

REMEMBER

Single-sided deafness, as mentioned in the previous section, can also be treated with a cochlear implant. While the overall goal of both types of devices is the same (allowing the person to hear and communicate better), the way that this is done is very different between the two devices: A CI device restores function to the affected side, whereas an osseointegrated hearing device just routes sound from the non-hearing to the hearing ear. Both approaches have different advantages and disadvantages, which an audiologist and ENT specializing in otology or neurotology can explain to you in greater depth.

4

Supporting Hearing Needs

IN THIS CHAPTER

» **Seeing the impact of hearing loss on relationships**

» **Understanding what people with hearing loss are experiencing**

» **Discovering strategies to improve communication and relationships for those with hearing loss**

» **Recognizing the hearing and communication needs of others**

» **Being aware of how to help someone with hearing loss**

Chapter 14

Helping Those with Hearing Loss

"It takes two to tango."

We know, we know . . . "two to tango" certainly isn't a novel phrase, but it captures a lot of the dimensions of hearing and communication. A conversation, like the tango, takes at least two people, and each person's role is essential in making the conversation (or dance) go smoothly. When one person is struggling a bit (whether forgetting some dance steps or having hearing loss), their partner can help things still go smoothly if the partner knows what they're doing!

If you would like to help someone who has hearing issues, this chapter is here to reveal important and helpful strategies to use when communicating with someone with hearing loss.

Noting How Hearing Loss Influences Relationships

Most of us have probably heard that effective communication is essential to all relationships.

Well, you can probably begin to guess from your own personal experience or observing others what can happen when hearing loss begins to interfere with the spoken conversations that make up much of your day-to-day communication. Friction in these daily conversations can arise from many sources. Here are the common ones we hear about:

» The communication partner (the person trying to communicate with someone with hearing loss) becoming irritated when the individual with hearing loss seems to frequently misunderstand or ignore them

» The individual with hearing loss blaming the communication partner for always "mumbling" and not speaking clearly

» The individual with hearing loss getting tired with struggling to hear and emotionally checking out or refusing to go to social gatherings with their communication partner

» The communication partner feeling like they have to be the translator for the individual with hearing loss in settings such as social gatherings, stores, and healthcare visits

The *most* important thing to note about these examples is that they are all *addressable* with the right communication strategies! This chapter details communication strategies for the communication partner. Complementary strategies for the individual with hearing loss are explained in Chapter 8.

Understanding Hearing Loss from the Other Side

At some point, you've probably experienced the difficulty of trying to communicate with someone on a cell-phone call with poor reception. If so, this experience reflects what it sounds like to hear with hearing loss — the exception being, of course, that for the individual with hearing loss, everything sounds like this and not just when the person is on a call. The extent to how garbled and muffled the sound is depends on the severity of the individual's hearing loss.

Emotions that often accompany hearing loss

Being on a crackly phone call for a few minutes is annoying. Now imagine the feelings that come with being on a crackly phone call *every single time* you talk to another person. This is what it's like to live with hearing loss. And a wide range of emotions accompany the day-to-day struggle.

While some individuals may adapt well to communicating with hearing loss, others may respond with frustration, anger, or resentment, or constantly blame others for mumbling all the time. Some may withdraw from social situations or sit silently in the corner at social events.

Some individuals respond to their hearing problems by taking the opposite tack and instead try to dominate conversations at social gatherings. Why's this, you may ask? Well, because if you're the person who's doing most of the talking, you know what's actually being said!

How individuals emotionally cope with and respond to having hearing loss is influenced by

>> Their personality and how they respond to life stressors

>> Their previous life experiences

>> Their understanding of hearing and hearing loss

>> External factors that affect the quality of the sounds that the person is trying to hear (such as background noise)

REMEMBER

While people with hearing loss can't necessarily change their personality or previous life experiences to affect how they respond to a hearing loss, you can use the strategies in this chapter to influence how well people in your life with hearing loss understand their hearing (and hence feel empowered to do something about it) and how you can change other external factors that affect how well they can hear.

Realizing hearing aids don't cure hearing loss

A common refrain we hear from our patients' family members is something along the lines of "We bought Mom $4,000 hearing aids and she still can't hear."

HOW EYEGLASSES DIFFER FROM HEARING AIDS

The question often comes up of why eyeglasses seem to completely correct vision problems, but hearing aids don't do the same for hearing loss. The answer stems from the fact that the cause of most vision problems is completely difference from the cause of hearing loss.

Vision problems most often stem from refractive errors, meaning that light is not being focused clearly onto the retina (the part of the eye that sends the signal to the brain similar to the role of the cochlea in the ear). If these light rays are focused properly onto the retina with the use of eyeglasses or contact lenses, voilà! The person can see perfectly again.

Note there are some analogous problems in vision that are similar to hearing loss, including glaucoma and macular degeneration, which damage the retina. In these cases, as you may expect, glasses can't fix the problem, similar to the way a hearing aid can't fix hearing loss.

This statement is usually spoken in exasperation as communication challenges persist despite the amount of money spent on the problem. It's important to remember that the hearing loss that occurs over time we address in this book can't be fixed with hearing aids any more than a prosthetic leg can fix an amputated leg.

A hearing aid can certainly make communication easier, but it still depends on the individual employing different communication strategies (see Chapter 8), having realistic expectations of how a hearing aid can help but not fix hearing loss, and optimizing external factors that can improve the sound quality of what the person hears.

Discovering How to Be a Good Communication Partner

Strategies to be a good communication partner focus on how you can improve the quality of sound to make it easier for your partner to understand you. A clearer and better-quality sound signal can help compensate for the detrimental effects of hearing loss (see Chapters 3 and 8). The following sections detail how you can help.

Move close and speak face-to-face

Sound loudness and quality both drop off quickly with increasing distance from the speaker, so get closer — ideally at arm's length. In particular, in certain rooms with high ceilings or lots of hard surfaces, there can be a lot of echo or reverberation, which can rapidly degrade the quality of your voice if you're too far from the person you're speaking with.

You want to be face-to-face with the person you're speaking with as well. For example, at a restaurant or a meeting table, communicating is easier when you're across from the person you want to speak with rather than side by side, despite your being close to the person in both situations. Being face-to-face allows the other person to see the visual cues of your lip movements and facial expressions, and these additional cues are hugely helpful for allowing the brain to quickly translate sounds into meaning.

Repeat and reword

If someone doesn't hear what you say, the tendency is to just repeat what you just said, perhaps a little louder. For example, you may say, "Where should we go out for dinner tonight?" and when you get a blank stare or a "huh" or "what" response, you just repeat the question.

This is natural and in general works well since the repetition may simply allow the listener to catch a few of the words that were missed the first time.

TIP

If you get a huh/what again after the second repetition, though, avoid repeating the exact same utterance. Instead, rephrase or reword your original question. For example, say something like "Which restaurant do you want to try this evening?"

The statement is similar to the original phrase ("Where should we go out for dinner tonight?") but the introduction of similar but different phrases (in this example, "restaurant" and "evening" instead of "dinner" and "tonight") can better clue in the listener to what you're saying if the original message isn't getting across because of hearing loss. This rephrasing allows the listener's brain to further narrow down and pinpoint the exact meaning of what you're trying to say.

Speak slowly and clearly

REMEMBER

This may seem obvious, but people often have a tendency to shout when not being heard. Instead, slowing down the pace of your speech is the most important thing to do. Speaking slightly louder certainly helps as well, but often if your voice is too loud, it becomes more distorted and affects the quality of sound.

Speaking slowly and clearly is so important with hearing loss because the listener's brain is always getting a slightly more garbled version of what you're actually saying. Because of this garbling, the brain can take just a bit longer to decode and process the sound signal into actual meaning. If you're speaking too fast, the listener can still be stuck on figuring out your first sentence when you're already on your third sentence.

Get your partner's attention before speaking

This may seem like another obvious strategy, but it's easily forgotten about, particularly at home. When you want to say something to your partner, even when your partner may be in the next room of the house, you may just say it without first ensuring that your partner is ready to listen to you. For example, you may launch into a conversation about plans for the day when, in fact, your partner was paying attention to the TV or focused on another task and never even initially heard you.

TIP

When possible, wait to begin conversations until you're in the same room, with any background noise minimized, and you clearly know you have your partner's attention. You can physically tap the person on the shoulder, stand face-to-face, or get spoken confirmation that your partner is listening to you. These simple, common-sense steps can go a long way toward minimizing friction with communication.

Choose the right environments for conversations

Rooms that are smaller, with lower ceilings, and lots of soft surfaces (for example, carpeted floors, drapes, and upholstered furniture) can make communication a lot easier. These factors all reduce the amount of reverberation or echoing of sound in the room and can be taken into consideration if you're ever faced with the choice of picking a restaurant or meeting room. In any situation, you'll also want to minimize any ongoing background noise (for example, turning down any music or turning off a noisy air conditioner).

Using technologies to help communication

There are some everyday technologies that can be used to improve communication with a person who has hearing loss. These are also covered in other parts of the book (Chapters 8 and 12) but are quickly summarized here again for reference:

>> Calls made over Voice over Internet Protocol (VOIP) services such as FaceTime, Google Meet, Line, Microsoft Teams, Skype, WhatsApp, and Zoom will all provide a clearer and better quality sound signal than a conventional phone call made over a landline phone or cellular phone.

>> Videocalls are even better than audio-only calls because they allow for both auditory and visual cues in communication. These additional visual cues make it much, much easier to understand what is being spoken.

>> Live automated captioning is now available on many technology platforms, including Microsoft Teams and Zoom, and is built into software used for presentations like Microsoft PowerPoint. Consider turning these captioning services on to allow everyone listening to have access to these additional communication cues.

Figuring Out Hearing and Communication Needs

You may wonder how to know which of the strategies in this chapter you need to use and whether, in fact, your communication partner needs you to use them. There are a couple of ways to approach this.

Noticing non-verbal cues

The first approach, known as subjective impression, is to notice — based on the back and forth of the conversation — whether the listener is in fact understanding you. This is sometimes obvious based on how the person verbally responds but not always depending on how well you know the person. Non-verbal cues can often give the best hints. These non-verbal cues include

>> The listener looks slightly puzzled or quizzical as you're speaking.

>> The listener stares intently at your lips or face as you're speaking.

>> The listener's non-verbal acknowledgments of what you're saying (such as a nod of the head or smile) are slightly delayed relative to what you're saying.

If you're noticing any of the signs mentioned here when talking to someone, there's a good chance that person is having trouble hearing you. In these cases, you'll want to make sure to follow the communication strategies detailed in this chapter.

Using the hearing number as a guide

Another, more objective way of understanding your communication partner's needs is to know their hearing number. The hearing number is calculated from a person's audiogram and reflects how loud speech sounds have to be for the person to reliably hear them (see Chapters 5 and 7).

REMEMBER

A general rule of thumb to remember is that the higher your partner's hearing number is, the greater the severity of hearing loss and the more communication strategies you need to use on a daily basis to ensure communication goes smoothly.

If your partner's hearing number is

>> **0 to 25:** This is generally considered the normal range of hearing, but as the hearing number gets into the 20s, start focusing on getting close and speaking face-to-face.

>> **26 to 40:** You definitely want to be getting close and face-to-face routinely, particularly whenever there's a lot of background noise (for example, being at a busy coffee shop).

>> **41 to 60:** Start adding in at least one or more of the other communication strategies and be strategic about the settings in which you communicate.

>> **Greater than 60:** You definitely want to use all the communication strategies detailed in this chapter and avoid noisy environments when the goal is effective communication.

Supporting People on Their Hearing Care Journey

Everyone approaches the challenges of communicating with people who have hearing loss in their own way. Some ignore it, others embrace it, and for others, it's a long process of education and awareness before anything is considered. The goal is that we all just want to be able to communicate as effortlessly as possible in all settings. Here are a few critical things to keep in mind to best support others in your life:

>> **Follow the communication strategies explained in this chapter.** These are some of the most important things you can do on a daily basis to optimize effective communication with virtually anyone (irrespective of their level of hearing).

>> **Optimize your communication environment.** Pick environments that are easier for communication (such as smaller rooms with lots of soft surfaces to reduce reverberation, little or no background noise, and better lighting).

>> **Knowledge is power.** Be aware of the content we cover in this book about how hearing works and the different communication strategies and technologies available to help.

>> **Don't accept the struggle.** Encourage those in your life who have hearing loss to look into treatment. They don't have to simply accept and live with hearing loss. They can be empowered to make positive changes. Being able to effectively communicate and engage with the world around us is absolutely fundamental to our health and well-being and cannot be ignored.

Chapter **15**

Paying for Hearing Care

P aying for hearing care can seem daunting, but it can be managed. In this chapter, we take you through the ins and outs of paying for hearing health. What are the costs involved? What's covered by insurance? We then look specifically at the cost of hearing aids, what that cost covers, where to purchase them, and options like paying through a health savings account or flexible savings account and getting them from charitable organizations.

If you're concerned about your hearing, don't let the cost get in your way of seeking help. We can't say this enough: Addressing hearing loss is one step you can take to keep healthy, vital, and engaged in life. And fortunately, except for hearing aids, which we cover later in this chapter, some costs of hearing care are covered by insurance.

Paying for Hearing Services

Hearing services are the critical testing, evaluation, and treatment services typically provided by an audiologist or hearing instrument specialist as well as the medical and surgical services provided by an ear, nose, and throat (ENT) doctor when needed.

Hearing testing

Diagnostic hearing testing is most commonly done by an audiologist, and these diagnostic tests when done by an audiologist are generally covered by standard health insurance plans.

While the test is covered, some insurance plans (including traditional Medicare plans) may require a referral from your primary care doctor. Other insurance plans don't require this referral, and you can schedule an appointment directly with an audiologist.

WARNING

In contrast, you may also find that many retail hearing aid outlets offer free hearing tests and evaluations where you can make an appointment or just walk in. These retail clinics exist solely to sell and service hearing aids, and a "free" hearing test in this regard is being done as a precursor to what the retail outlet hopes will be a hearing aid sale. There's nothing necessarily wrong with these tests, but just be forewarned that the free hearing test will likely come with a pitch to sell you hearing aids. At these retail outlets, the person doing the hearing test may be an audiologist or a hearing instrument specialist (see Chapter 7).

Medical and surgical evaluation

Evaluation by an ENT doctor for any medical or surgical conditions of the ear (see Chapters 3 and 13) is routinely covered by health insurance plans, although your insurance plan may require a referral from your primary care doctor. During this evaluation, an ENT will gather a medical history and conduct an examination of your ears.

Some types of hearing loss can be treated with surgery, and in most cases, these surgeries and surgically implantable hearing devices (such as cochlear implants for severe hearing loss) are covered by insurance, but some insurance plans may have very specific criteria for when these implantable devices would be covered.

Hearing rehabilitative support services

An audiologist provides education and rehabilitative services to help you under-stand what may be the best hearing options for you, to explain how to use various communication strategies, and to provide support for hearing technologies, such as hearing aids and cochlear implants. A hearing instrument specialist provides a much narrower set of services focused only on supporting hearing aid use.

Unfortunately for the consumer, these important services are almost never covered by insurance plans (except in the case of cochlear implants). As a result, most hearing care professionals will provide these services only if you buy a hearing aid from the provider, and these services are "bundled" into the overall cost of the hearing aid.

This bundling of hearing care services with a hearing aid sale is not good for consumers. For example, if you were interested in buying your own over-the-counter (OTC) hearing aid, you may still need a hearing care professional's guidance as to which devices to consider and how to best use these devices to address your listening needs.

Likewise, some individuals with trouble hearing don't need a hearing aid and would simply benefit from seeing an audiologist to learn about the best communication strategies and non-hearing-aid hearing technologies to use routinely (such as smartphone-based hearing amplifiers and captioned phones; see Chapter 12).

In both of these cases, most hearing care professionals aren't yet used to offering such professional services unbundled from the sale of a hearing aid. In the past, unbundling wasn't necessary because consumers could buy hearing aids only from a hearing care professional. The imminent availability of OTC hearing aids in the United States by the end of 2022, however, is forcing hearing care professionals to adapt and change.

TIP

If you want the help of a hearing professional to understand and address your hearing but don't want to necessarily buy a hearing aid from them, ask in advance if the provider offers hearing care services unbundled from the sale of a hearing aid. Not all do yet, but this will increasingly change over the next few years.

BUNDLING DEVICE AND SERVICE LIMITS THE EFFECTIVENESS OF HEARING CARE

Bundling refers to the practice of combining the cost of the hearing aid with the hearing care professional services. The overwhelming majority of hearing aid clinics use this method, but it has contributed to creating a stiff and rigid hearing care system that, in our experience, only meets the needs of a narrow group of hearing aid users.

Bundling creates a lack of transparency that is bad for everyone involved. By combining everything into one price, consumers don't know what they have paid for and may fail

(continued)

(continued)

to take full advantage of the prepaid services. On the other side, bundling masks the importance of the professional services by putting the spotlight on the hearing aid. The result is some view hearing care professionals as hearing aid salespersons rather than as practitioners of hearing care. Lastly, bundling completely anonymizes the manufacturers and doesn't incentivize them to offer competitive pricing to consumers.

Hearing care professionals, particularly audiologists, cannot practice to their full skillset in the bundled care model. Audiologists spend four years obtaining a clinical doctorate degree with countless classroom and internship hours spent focusing on a full range of hearing care and audiologic rehabilitation services. But some are disappointed to find the reality that the bundled model incentivizes hearing aid sales rather than offering a full range of services.

For the consumer, bundling means hearing care is an all-or-none endeavor. Either you buy a hearing aid and access the services of a professional or you're on your own. There are no options for appointments unrelated to the hearing aid, such as a counseling session to offer guidance on coping with hearing loss, a visit to go over communication strategies, or a rehabilitation auditory training session. This leaves millions of adults with hearing loss unable to get the services that meet them where they are in their hearing care journey.

Bundling also ties the consumer to a single hearing aid clinic for the lifetime of the hearing aid. With the practice of paying for all services up front, it is near impossible to make a smooth transition to a new hearing care professional without buying a new hearing aid. What happens when someone with hearing aids moves? Either they end up paying for services they already paid for once with a new hearing care professional or, in some cases, the new hearing care professional eats the cost of their time. Someone loses in that situation.

Unbundling will likely start in the United States with the new OTC hearing aid category. Consumers will be able to choose a la carte services or even bundled service plan options for those who prefer it — the key is a future where there is greater transparency in the costs of the hearing aids versus professional hearing support services.

Breaking Down Hearing Aid Costs

Hearing aids can cost thousands of dollars. By some estimates, getting a pair of hearing aids in the United States can, on average, set you back $4,000! The cost for a pair of hearing aids ranges from the low $1,000s all the way up to $7,000–$8,000. For many people, that may mean a simple pair of hearing aids is their third largest material purchase in life after a house and car.

Why the heck are they so expensive? The simple answer is that when you buy a set of hearing aids, you're paying for both the hearing aids and the services that the hearing care professional is providing to program, adjust, and teach you how to use the hearing aid (for more information, see the sidebar "Why are hearing aids so expensive?" later in this chapter).

This lack of transparency with how hearing aids are sold is really bad and prevents consumers from understanding what they're paying for. Fortunately, with the imminent availability of OTC hearing aids that you'll be able to purchase without going through a professional, hearing care providers will increasingly be unbundling their costs so you'll know exactly you're paying for. At the same time, the increased competition in the hearing aid market that will come with OTC hearing aids means that the costs of all hearing aids will likely also decrease over time.

At present, most hearing aids are purchased out-of-pocket. Some private insurance plans offer some coverage, but many do not; check your plan. Traditional Medicare does not cover hearing aids.

The following sections cover different ways to pay for hearing aids.

Weighing out-of-pocket-options

Recall that when you're buying prescription hearing aids from a professional that you're paying for both the hearing aids and the professional's services to test, program, and fit the hearing aids plus the time they spend working with you to ensure that you're communicating well with the hearing aid.

Prescription hearing aids can be purchased out-of-pocket through any of the following channels:

>> Audiologists working independently or in a hospital or ENT practice

>> Retail hearing aid clinics owned directly by a hearing aid manufacturer and typically staffed by a hearing instrument specialist (rather than an audiologist)

>> Big box stores such as Costco and Sam's Club

>> Internet or online sales

Given that prescription hearing aids purchased through these channels cost thousands of dollars, many of these channels offer consumers the option of using some type of payment plan.

The Costco effect

Over the past decade, Costco has increasingly been accounting for more and more of the hearing aids sold in the United States and is now the second largest provider of hearing aids in the country after the U.S. Veterans Administration. By virtue of scale (Costco can command a very low wholesale price from the hearing aid manufacturers), it has been able to substantially bring down the price of hearing aids while also establishing strict protocols to ensure that hearing aids are properly fit and programmed by the hearing care professionals working for Costco. At the time of printing, a pair of store-branded Costco hearing aids produced by the largest manufacturer of hearing aids was advertised at about $1,400, inclusive of all hearing care services and a six-month refundable trial period.

Online sales of hearing aids

Even prior to the release of OTC hearing aids, you could find hearing aids over the internet. Hearing aids purchased this way generally don't come with any related support services. If you're considering buying hearing aids online, thoroughly research what you're getting. Up to now, the U.S. Food and Drug Administration (FDA) hasn't regulated hearing aids purchased online to ensure they are safe and effective for use directly by the consumer. With the release of FDA regulations for OTC hearing aids expected by the end of 2022, it should be much easier and safer to buy a hearing aid online.

Other companies are also now beginning to offer hybrid services (for example, listenlively.com) where the hearing aids are purchased over the internet, but the company offers extensive virtual support services via video calls with a hearing care provider to help the consumer learn how to use the hearing aid.

Checking on insurance coverage options for hearing aids

Hearing aids are the most common technology option for treating the majority of hearing losses. A few insurance options exist as detailed in the next sections. In considering some of the main coverage options for hearing aids, keep in mind that the information given is specifically in reference to hearing aid coverage options for adults with hearing loss. Pediatric hearing loss is managed completely differently from both a medical and audiological perspective, and insurance plans also have completely different hearing coverage policies for children versus adults.

TIP

The Hearing Loss Association of America website covers various options for covering the cost of hearing aids at `www.hearingloss.org/hearing-help/financial-assistance/`.

SO WHERE SHOULD I BUY HEARING AIDS?

If you don't have insurance or VA coverage, you may be asking at this point which of the out-of-pocket hearing aid channels may be best for you. There's not necessarily a right answer to this question, but as a general rule of thumb, we suggest the following:

- If you have a more substantial hearing loss, have a complicated medical history for your hearing loss (that is, not just a gradual hearing loss over time) or complex hearing and communication needs (such as working in noisy environments), or would like a comprehensive evaluation of your hearing and communication needs, you should start with an audiologist who works independently or with an ENT practice since you may also need a medical evaluation.

- For a slowly progressive hearing loss in both ears that has come on gradually over many years, you can consider trying a big box store. Costco has become the largest private retailer of hearing aids in the United States and is consistently ranked highly by Consumer Reports. Its fully refundable six-month trial period is a risk-free way to see if the hearing aids and your experience with the hearing care professional at Costco are working for you.

- Retail hearing aid clinics can be okay, but our impression is that there's so much variability in the level and quality of service and technology that it's hard for us to make a recommendation. At best, you'll get a highly trained hearing care provider who will prioritize making sure your hearing and communication needs are being met. At worst, you'll encounter a retail sales experience where you get the impression that someone is trying to sell you the most expensive hearing aid you're willing to buy regardless of whether you need it and with a questionable scientific or clinical basis for whether the more expensive hearing aid is even better.

- The online purchase model is in a lot of flux now as OTC hearing aids are slated to enter the market in late 2022. Once OTC hearing aids are formally out there, buying an FDA-regulated OTC hearing aid online will be fine for mild to moderate hearing loss. Until then, you have to approach hearing aids sold online somewhat warily since many aren't regulated to ensure they're safe and effective to use without the assistance of hearing care providers. Some online companies offer internet sales coupled with lots of virtual support services. These may also be a reasonable option to try if you find that the hearing aid and cost meet your needs and budget.

Traditional Medicare

Traditional Medicare is the most common type of Medicare plan that the majority of adults 65 years and older (and other younger individuals who qualify for Medicare) have in the United States. Under traditional Medicare, while hearing diagnostic services provided by an audiologist are covered with a medical referral, any related hearing rehabilitative services or hearing aids are not.

Medicare Advantage Plans

Medicare Advantage plans are private insurance plans that people over age 65 can select over traditional Medicare coverage. While traditional Medicare plans don't cover hearing aids, a Medicare Advantage plan might.

The types of benefits, however, can vary widely. Some Medicare Advantage plans offer a fixed reimbursement amount (for example, $2,000 every three years) for hearing aids while others specifically refer you to a third-party hearing coverage insurance network. These hearing networks are often a subsidiary of a hearing aid manufacturer that has its own retail shops or contracts with certain hearing providers to offer its hearing aids.

WARNING

This type of "coverage" through a third-party hearing network in many cases may just be for some sort of discount off of the regular cost of a hearing aid, and patients still incur substantial out-of-pocket costs in the thousands of dollars. In many cases, you may be better off considering all your options before automatically assuming the hearing aid benefit from your Medicare Advantage plan offers any real benefit or is a good deal for your money.

Private insurance

There's a lot of variability in whether private (typically employer-sponsored) health insurance plans cover hearing aids. When they do offer coverage, their plan offerings will be similar to the Medicare Advantage plans explained earlier since Medicare Advantage plans are essentially the same as private insurance (but subsidized in part by the government).

Medicaid

Medicaid health insurance plans are government-subsidized insurance plans for low-income people meeting specific income criteria. These plans are managed at the state level, and coverage benefits can vary state by state. Some state-level Medicaid plans now include coverage for hearing aids that in many cases don't involve any out-of-pocket costs.

The main issue with this coverage, though, is that depending on the state, the Medicaid plan's reimbursement levels for the audiologist to provide a hearing aid may be so low that many audiologists can't afford to participate because they would be losing money every time they saw a patient. At one extreme, some state Medicaid plans may reimburse the audiologist for the wholesale cost of the hearing aid but provide little to no reimbursement for the hours of time that the audiologist spends working with the patient.

For this reason, you'll sometimes find that only audiologists at large hospitals, nonprofit hearing clinics, or academic medical centers participate in Medicaid plans.

WHY ARE HEARING AIDS SO EXPENSIVE?

When purchasing a hearing aid from a hearing care provider, the cost of the hearing aid generally includes all the services that the audiologist or hearing instrument specialist is providing, which include

- "Free" hearing tests (you're actually paying for the test somewhere in the total cost)
- Counseling and education in using the hearing aid
- Programming of the hearing aid
- Continued care, maintenance, and support

The audiologist services are usually covered for the lifetime of the hearing aid, so you're essentially paying in advance for services that you may or may not use. A warranty from the manufacturer is included in the price as well and usually covered repairs and a limited number of replacements for two to three years after the purchase.

At the same time, you're also paying for the actual cost of the hearing aids, which reflects their wholesale cost. One key issue is that the wholesale price that hearing care providers pay can vary widely by how good of a deal they got, whether they have some type of exclusive deal with the manufacturer, and whether they are directly employed by the manufacturer in a manufacturer-owned retail clinic.

The result? The cost of hearing aids varies widely. In most cases, in a bundled hearing aid package, the wholesale hearing aid cost may represent only 25 percent to 50 percent of what you're paying, according to some experts. So if, for example, if you pay $4,000 for a set of hearing aids, the actual wholesale cost of the hearing aids may have only been $1,000-$2,000. Keep in mind, though, that not all hearing care professionals get such good wholesale prices depending on the volume of hearing aids they purchase from a manufacturer.

Looking to the future: Over-the-counter hearing aids

The expected release of FDA regulations for over-the-counter hearing aids by the end of 2022 will finally allow consumers to purchase FDA-approved and regulated hearing aids at retail stores. These devices are designed to be safe and effective without the need for professional services. Researchers expect that the cost of hearing aids will decrease dramatically as this market develops, with more companies (particularly consumer technology companies already making wearable hearing technologies) entering the hearing aid market. Until these FDA regulations, slated for late summer or fall 2022, come out, hearing aids can't legally be sold over-the-counter to consumers in the United States.

At the time of this publication, it's still unknown how insurance companies will consider covering or reimbursing for OTC hearing aids.

Tapping into Veterans Administration benefits

The Veterans Administration (VA) is the country's largest provider of hearing aids. If you're qualified to receive VA benefits, you may be able to get all your hearing care needs, including hearing aids and hearing care services, provided to you at no charge depending on the severity of your hearing loss and whether it is connected to your military service. Specific policies for whether hearing aids and related services are covered based on your military service vary widely depending on your local VA hospital. If you qualify for VA health benefits based on your prior military service, check with your local VA to find out whether you qualify for hearing care coverage.

Seeking charitable foundations

Various charitable foundations can provide subsidized or low-cost hearing aids if you qualify, which is typically based on your income and other financial considerations. You may have to fill out a lot of paperwork and jump through some hoops, but this option may be worth investigating if you qualify. A great up-to-date resource that lists these charitable foundations is the website of the Hearing Loss Association of America — hearingloss.org/hearing-help/financial-assistance.

Using health savings and flexible spending accounts

Hearing aids are considered medical devices and can typically be paid for using funds from a Health Savings Account (HSA) or a Flexible Spending Account, if you've established one. These accounts allow you to contribute pre-tax dollars into an account fund that can be used to cover eligible medical expenses (however, for HSAs, once you enroll in Medicare, you are no longer able to make contributions).

Chapter **16**

Your Rights as Someone with Hearing Loss

A lot of this book focuses directly on your individual hearing: testing, treatment, communication strategies, and more. But we live in a complex society, and your hearing experience may also depend on barriers that are beyond your control. It's important to consider your rights as someone with hearing loss in our society.

In this chapter, we take a brief look into the history of disability and hearing loss and introduce the social model of disability as a means to view rights and accommodations in society. We then cover the Americans with Disabilities Act and Social Security Disability Insurance, two major government programs that help people with severe or profound hearing loss, and we also give guidance on how you can advocate for hearing rights.

Looking into Disability and Hearing Loss

People with hearing loss have been subject to discrimination, stereotyping, and exclusion from education, employment, and social engagement. Fortunately, the disability community has led movements to remove barriers for people with hearing loss and provide accommodations to ensure access and engagement in society, including in public settings and the workplace. A prime example of these gains is the passage of the Americans with Disabilities Act in 1990. But there is still work to be done, and advocacy efforts continue to push for a more inclusive society.

How do you define disability?

Under some government programs, such as Social Security Disability Insurance, or civil rights laws like the Americans with Disabilities Act, hearing loss is an eligible "disability." The term disability, however, has a different meaning to different people. There is no one-size-fits-all definition, and whether someone identifies as disabled or not is a matter of personal perspective and values.

The World Health Organization and the Centers for Disease Control and Prevention broadly define a disability as "any condition of the body or mind that makes it more difficult for a person to do certain activities and interact with the world around them." Very specific terms are used to describe and define disability. They include the following:

>> **Impairment** refers to an individual's body functions or structures, or mental functioning. In the case of most hearing loss, this is the result of dysfunctional cells or other structures in the cochlea.

>> **Activity limitation** refers to the performance of specific actions, such as difficulty seeing, hearing, walking, or problem solving.

>> **Participation restrictions** refers to an inability to fully engage in normal daily activities such as work, social and recreational activities, and obtaining healthcare and preventive services.

How to follow a social model of disability

The way we look at things helps frame our decisions and future actions. In this section, we want to introduce the social model of disability to help you understand how the environment shapes your experience with hearing loss and why it is important to support actions to not only address your hearing loss on an individual level but also by helping to reshape the world around you into one that is hearing-loss friendly.

Disability, including hearing loss, has been viewed through multiple lenses over time. A traditional view of disability has been narrowly focused on only the medical model, which examines the impairment in the individual. So, in the case of hearing loss, the medical model focuses only on the inner ear and how to treat it. The medical model puts a lot of attention on how to treat the individual to help them function in society.

A more recent concept is the social model of disability that views disability as something that is imposed on an individual by society. Rather than focusing solely on the person's impairment, the social model of disability looks broadly at societal barriers holding back people with disabilities from thriving. The social model flips the narrative from a narrow focus on only impairment to a broad look at the individual's needs and goals in the context of their lifestyle and society.

Using the social model to approach your journey with hearing loss leads to better outcomes. In addition to any hearing technologies or communication strategies you adopt on your own, a holistic hearing care plan through the social model

>> Involves people in your network and educates them on accommodations for communication with hearing loss

>> Identifies barriers in your environment and develops solutions

>> Considers support groups for empowerment

>> Fosters self-advocacy for accommodations and access

>> Engages in person-centered care that aligns with your goals

>> Supports advocacy groups and public health measures in promoting efforts to create a more equal and accessible society

REMEMBER

Something important to always consider when discussing societal barriers for adults with disabilities is that breaking down these barriers doesn't negatively affect other people. In fact, many of the accommodations and design considerations intended to break down barriers for people with disabilities end up benefiting everyone. Examples include accessible captioning, curb cuts in the sidewalk, and the use of ramps in building codes. Everyone can benefit from these considerations.

Understanding the Role of the Americans with Disabilities Act

The Americans with Disabilities Act (ADA), passed in 1990, is a civil rights law aimed at providing protections from discrimination against people with disabilities. The law applies to employment, public places, public services and activities, and telecommunication, among other areas of society.

REMEMBER

The ADA does not define specific disabilities and instead uses broad language to consider disability as "physical or mental impairments" that limit an individual's life activities. There are no requirements based on the severity of the impairment or even whether or not the impairment is permanent.

Discouraging disability discrimination in the workplace

Under the ADA, employers with more than 15 employees must provide equal opportunity and accessibility for people with disabilities to engage in work-related activities and benefits. Employers must provide reasonable accommodations for people with disabilities to engage in work. Specific to hearing loss, these may include the provision of an amplified headset, captioned telephone, preferential seating in meetings, and captioning and Communication Access Real-Time Translation (CART) services during meetings (see Chapter 12). The ADA also prohibits discrimination in things like hiring, promotions, and pay.

TIP

Visit the U.S. Equal Employment Opportunity Commission at www.eeoc.gov to find out more about reasonable accommodations and the process for enforcing the Americans with Disabilities Act in the workplace.

Accessibility and accommodations in public

The ADA promotes accessibility and appropriate accommodations in broader parts of society beyond employment. Specifically, the ADA supports accessibility and engagement in government-supported programs and activities such as these:

>> Public education

>> Government recreation centers

>> Public libraries

>> Government-sponsored health services centers

>> Voting and other political activities

>> Public transportation

In addition, the ADA applies to private entities where the public gathers, including, but not limited to

>> Restaurants

>> Cinemas and theaters

>> Museums

>> Convention centers

>> Hospitals, doctor's offices, and other healthcare facilities

>> Recreational facilities like zoos or sports stadiums

Examples of accessibility in government services and public places specific to hearing loss may be the provision of appropriate amplification in school settings, captioning services during a political event or in a theater, or amplified personal audio systems in museums or libraries.

Focusing on telephones and television

The ADA also specifically requires telecommunications services like telephones and television services to be accessible. This aspect of the ADA is overseen by the U.S. Federal Communications Commission and includes the provision of closed captioning on television and services to support captioned telephones.

TIP

For more information on hearing loops to support accessibility in public places and captioned telephones, see Chapter 12. You can also visit www.ada.gov to find more details on the Americans with Disabilities Act.

Navigating the Social Security Administration Disability Benefits

While the ADA provides a legal basis for anti-discrimination, what happens if you're in the incredibly stressful situation of being unable to work due to your hearing loss? Adults with severe or profound hearing loss that affects their ability to work may be eligible for Social Security Administration (SSA) disability benefits.

Public programs that provide disability insurance play a key role in building a supportive society. Some form of public disability insurance in the United States has existed since the 1956 amendments to the Social Security Act. The SSA oversees the largest disability benefits programs in the United States. There are two main programs related to disability at SSA:

>> **Social Security Disability Insurance** (SSDI) provides monthly disability benefits to qualified individuals "who can't work because they have a medical condition that's expected to last at least one year or result in death."

>> **Supplemental Security Income** (SSI) is a needs-based supplemental income program that can apply to people with disabilities with limited income and resources.

Adults with severe or profound hearing loss can collect both SSDI and SSI at the same time but each program has very specific intentions. SSDI is intended for when a condition prevents the ability to work regardless of taxable income and requires that a person has paid into Social Security for a certain period. SSI is needs-based with taxable income limits for qualification but no previous work requirements.

WARNING

Collecting both SSDI and SSI at the same time may affect SSI payments because it is dependent on income levels.

Determining hearing loss for Social Security disability benefits

If you're reading this chapter, you're thinking about Social Security benefits in terms of hearing loss. In addition to the criteria in the previous section, the SSA has very specific criteria of severe or profound hearing loss that meets SSI and SSDI eligibility.

WARNING

The following information includes some technical terms for hearing exams and definitions. The SSA uses strict criteria to define hearing loss, which differs from other organizations, and we want to present that here to you. See Chapter 7 for breakdowns of hearing professionals and hearing assessments and Chapter 13 for more information on medical evaluations of the ear and cochlear implants.

Evaluating hearing loss

Since the SSA uses a very specific set of criteria, it can be complex to navigate how it defines hearing loss. As of the publication of this book, a hearing evaluation for SSA should include the following:

- A medical exam performed by a licensed otolaryngologist

- A hearing exam performed by a licensed audiologist

  The hearing exam must include tests referred to as pure-tone air- and bone-conduction audiometry, speech reception threshold, and word recognition threshold for each ear.

  The hearing exam must take place in a sound booth that meets the American National Standards Institute's (ANSI's) standards for hearing testing.

  The assessment should take place without a hearing aid, even if you normally wear one.

  The assessment for people with cochlear implants must include a speech test called the Hearing in Noise Test (HINT).

Defining hearing loss

The SSA standard definition of hearing loss for disability benefits differs depending on treatment.

TECHNICAL STUFF

- **For hearing loss not treated with a cochlear implant,** using general terms, the SSA requires a profound or greater *sensorineural hearing loss* (see Chapter 7) in an individual's better ear. Alternatively, regardless of the level of hearing using pure-tone audiometry (see Chapter 7), the SSA considers those with a very poor ability to repeat words presented at loud but not uncomfortable levels to have disabling hearing loss.

  The technical definition of hearing loss is either of the following:

  - An average of the air conduction audiometry thresholds at 500, 1,000, and 2,000 Hz greater than or equal to 90 decibels in the better hearing ear without any bone-conduction thresholds better than 60 decibels

  - A word recognition test score of less than 40 percent in the better ear

  Check out Chapter 7 for help on understanding test results.

- **For hearing loss that is treated with a cochlear implant,** an individual is considered to have a disabling hearing loss for the first year following surgery. After the first year, the determination is based on a speech test (HINT) score of 60 percent or less. This score means that even while wearing the cochlear implant, an individual struggles to understand speech when it is presented with some background noise.

Considering Claims for SSDI

The SSA considers many factors in determining an SSDI claim. They include information on your age and work history, income, a medical and hearing evaluation, and the nature of your work.

Age and work history

To determine whether you qualify for SSDI, the SSA first looks at your age and work history. Most people working in the United States pay a certain percentage of federal taxes for the SSA program. To qualify for SSDI, you must have paid into the program for a certain amount of time. The time varies based on the age at which you become disabled. The older you are when you become disabled, the more time you need to have worked to qualify for disability insurance.

Substantial gainful activity

Eligibility for SSDI is also affected by what the SSA calls *substantial gainful activity*. This is based on your work activity and any income you derive from it. These both need to be below certain levels for an individual to qualify for SSDI.

Medical evaluation

The SSA uses the results of a medical evaluation to guide its decision on determining a disability insurance claim. The SSA has its own guide to disability considerations called the Blue Book that includes specific criteria for evaluation and definition of various impairments, including hearing loss (see the earlier section, "Defining hearing loss" for details on how the SSA defines it).

TIP

For more details on the SSA Blue Book visit: www.ssa.gov/disability/professionals/bluebook/AdultListings.htm.

Nature of work and accommodations

The SSA examines the duties needed to perform your job and uses the results of a medical evaluation to determine whether your disability prevents you from performing any of those duties. The SSA also looks at whether, based on the medical evaluation, you could perform other work.

Additionally, the SSA considers whether reasonable accommodations have been implemented, or should be attempted, and factors this into a decision. For people with hearing loss, for example, you may be provided with an amplified headset to use with your phone in the office to perform your duties.

Looking at Supplemental Security Income

When applying for SSI, you may also need to provide a medical evaluation as described previously. Unlike SSDI, applying for SSI does not depend on work history, contributions to Social Security through taxes, or substantial gainful activities. Instead, when applying for SSI, the main factor for eligibility is an income limit set by the SSA. This limits changes annually so check the SSA website, www.ssa.gov, for more info.

TIP

Unlike SSDI, SSI benefits vary from state to state, and some states will contribute additional payments to the federal SSI benefit.

Initiating a claim

TIP

The first step in the process of receiving disability benefits for both SSDI and SSI is to visit www.ssa.gov to initiate a claim. Just like many things in life, navigating SSA disability benefits can be a long process. Be prepared and be patient. The SSA has a lot of strict criteria to follow, and it may require lots of information and plenty of back and forth.

Advocating to Advance Your Hearing Rights

The Americans with Disabilities Act and Social Security Disability Insurance are just two of the many programs passed through the efforts of a large coalition of advocates. But there is more to be done.

Advocating for change

Public policy occurs at the federal, state, and local government levels in the United States, and getting involved at any level can help to advance the rights of people with hearing loss.

This can include a wide range of topics from big national initiatives to narrow local laws. At the federal level, you might, for example, support expanded Medicare coverage related to hearing aids. At the local level, you might support a city government bill providing funds for installing a hearing loop in city hall to improve access for people with hearing aids.

How can you get involved? Contact your representatives to show your support for legislation and provide supporting evidence for your position. Or you can raise money or organize events to support a specific cause.

TIP

To get more involved in advocating for the rights of people with hearing loss, visit the Hearing Loss Association of America's (HLAA's) website at www.hearingloss. org and check out the advocacy section to find a listing of local chapters near you.

Improving organization policy

Not all policy is government-based. Various employment, health, and public recreation settings could benefit from advocacy related to improving understanding and accommodations for hearing loss. Advocacy at this level involves contacting organizations and lending your expertise in guiding organizational policies for accommodating hearing loss.

You can advocate at this level in a number of ways:

>> Develop and distribute tool kits for employers on making accommodations, or quick reference guides for best-practice communication tips in healthcare settings.

>> Host a hearing loss awareness event in your community or workplace.

>> Sit on a committee to consider ways to improve access to auditory information for people with hearing loss at a local auditorium or museum.

5

The Part of Tens

Chapter **17**

Ten (Plus One) Considerations When Purchasing Hearing Aids

So, you're going to purchase hearing aids, either through a professional or over the counter (OTC), and you're looking for some guidance. Awesome. Let's start with the good news. Hearing aids come in many excellent styles from numerous brands and have a lot of useful accessories and features. Now for the bad news. Hearing aids come in many excellent styles from numerous brands and have a lot of useful accessories and features. Where to begin with so many options?

In this chapter, we walk you through the various designs, accessories, cost, and use considerations to help you decide which hearing aids are best for you. Our goal is to send you on your way prepared to purchase hearing aids.

REMEMBER

Before we get going, a quick reminder that OTC hearing aids are intended for only mild to moderate hearing loss in adults, while prescription hearing aids can address all degrees of hearing loss. Keep this in mind because the choice between OTC and prescription depends on your level of hearing loss.

Paying More Does Not Guarantee Better Outcomes

The more expensive, the better the hearing aids, right? No! In the current hearing aid market, it is a mistake to attribute higher cost to better technology or a guarantee of a better experience.

The path of how a hearing aid reaches a consumer is complicated. Only five hearing aid manufacturers dominate the entire prescription hearing aid market, and several either own their own hearing aid clinics or sign various exclusive distribution deals with hearing care professionals. Also, when you purchase a hearing aid, the professional services are often bundled into the price such that it isn't clear how much of the cost you're paying is for services versus the device. The result of the complex logistics and sales model is that the same hearing aid can be sold at vastly different prices, even just down the street.

The bottom line is that higher cost does not necessarily equal a better product.

Selecting from the Many Styles

Prescription and over-the-counter hearing aids come in different shapes and sizes. And, in fact, new innovation from OTC hearing aids may introduce entirely new styles in the coming years.

At the time of this book, there are two main types of hearing aids: in-the-ear (ITE) or behind-the-ear (BTE).

There are variations within the ITE and BTE hearing aid styles. ITEs come in much smaller sizes called completely-in-the-canal (CIC) hearing aids that are nearly invisible. BTE's visibility depends on the size of the earpiece that goes into the ear canal.

Figure 17-1 shows the general look of ITE and BTE hearing aids and how they sit in the ear. Many people assume the BTE is more noticeable, but you'll see in the images that the BTE sits behind the ear (hence the name) and is mostly hidden.

FIGURE 17-1:
Styles of hearing aids displayed in and out of the ear. On the left is a BTE hearing aid while an ITE hearing aid is displayed on the right.

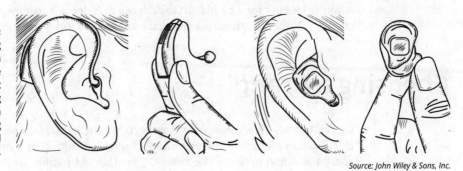

Source: John Wiley & Sons, Inc.

While the differences may only seem cosmetic, there are deeper considerations, such as:

>> Some ITE-style hearing aids are custom built, which requires taking an earmold impression.

WARNING

You can find at-home, do-it-yourself earmold impression kits, but proceed with caution. Without proper protection, the earmold impression material can get stuck in your ear canal or leave behind pieces stuck to your eardrum, requiring a medical professional to remove them. Make sure you're confident in the instructions and procedures if you are planning to use an at-home kit. We recommend seeing a professional for a custom ear impression.

>> The ITE design is much easier to insert into the ear for those with any stiffness or numbness in the hands as it involves just pushing it into the ear canal. It's even easier if it is custom built for your ears.

>> Very small ITE designs like the CIC limit the amount of space in the hearing aid and thus limit the maximum volume and features available — most notably, directionality.

>> The size of BTE hearing aids allow for compatibility with all features and complementary accessories.

TIP

In addition to the different styles available, there are numerous features to consider. While the availability of features vary from hearing aid to hearing aid and the needs of each individual is different, we suggest looking at features such as directionality to improve understanding speech in noise or automatic adjustment if you're looking for a hands-off experience that doesn't require you to manually change volume and programs yourself (see Chapter 10 for more on features).

Choosing a Brand

Currently, only five hearing aid manufacturers make over 90 percent of hearing aids. Each manufacturer owns multiple brands, resulting in a marketplace with dozens of brand options. The new OTC hearing aid market will see new brands enter the hearing aid market rapidly. Deciding on a specific brand may be different based on whether you're considering a prescription or OTC hearing aid.

In the prescription hearing aid market, the brand of hearing aid is usually determined by the professional's recommendation and comfort level with that brand. The major prescription hearing aid brands offer similar features and capabilities, albeit slightly different technology. Therefore, placing too much emphasis on brand may not be helpful for choosing prescription hearing aids.

WARNING

Don't pay too much attention to hearing aid rankings you might find in popular media for two reasons:

>> First, there is little science to the hearing aid rankings. They usually describe just a few features or someone's personal experience, but hearing care is highly individualized and what works for some won't work for others. The ranking systems can't take this into account.

>> Second, the rankings make it seem like one hearing aid is definitely better than the next, but the reality is that there is little difference between a hearing aid ranked first and another ranked tenth in meeting hearing needs. Remember: Hearing aids are held to some minimum standards by the U.S. Food and Drug Administration so the entire market is already curated to some degree.

For the newer category of over-the-counter hearing aids, the choice of brand may matter a little more based on your personal experience. While there are no established brands or companies in this market as of press time, if you like the sound quality of a certain tech company's headphones and that company now makes an OTC hearing aid, you may want to take that into consideration. Or you may consider a specific brand because you already own other audio products from that company and want your hearing aids to seamlessly connect.

REMEMBER

Hearing aids, both prescription and OTC, are regulated by the U.S. Food and Drug Administration and must meet minimum specifications to ensure they can address hearing loss. When a product calls itself a "hearing aid," that term already comes with some peace of mind that the technology is tested and approved.

Seeking Hearing Aids with Telecoils

Look for hearing aids that offer a telecoil. We can't recommend telecoils highly enough. These tiny parts of the hearing aid have been around for decades and keep proving themselves a reliable and useful feature. In short, a telecoil picks up on electromagnetic signals in the environment to give your hearing aids a direct connection to sound without amplifying extra background noise.

Telecoils work with telephones and at many public places such as museums, houses of worship, auditoriums, theaters and concert halls, airports, bus and train stations, and hospitals. Facilities install what are known as hearing loops that let hearing aid users get a direct signal from anywhere inside the building or room. Some telecoils will automatically detect and stream sound in these settings while other just require a simple press of a button to activate.

Powering Your Hearing Aid with Rechargeable Batteries

Our hearing aid patients used to complain all the time about the need to regularly purchase and change hearing aid batteries. Hearing aid manufacturers heeded this call and have introduced rechargeable hearing aids that provide enough juice for a full day of listening on a single charge. This saves you time and money by removing the need to buy disposable batteries. Even more important, rechargeable batteries eliminate the need to fiddle with the tiny battery compartment of hearing aids, making them easier to manipulate for those with less dexterity in their fingers.

TIP

Get into a good routine of charging your hearing aids overnight.

WARNING

There is always a flip side to every consideration. Rechargeable hearing aids require, well, charging. If you are worried about your ability to build the right routine to charge your hearing aids every night, disposable batteries may be a better choice for you. Just remember to carry extra batteries so you can quickly replace them when your hearing aid runs out of power.

Deciding on Open or Closed Fit

When researching your hearing aid options, whether OTC or prescription, you may see language around "open" and "closed" fitting or domes. This refers to whether the earpiece of the hearing aid that goes into your ear has some holes in it or not. Figure 17-2 shows an open and closed dome.

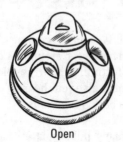
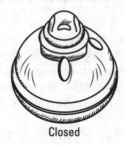

Open   Closed

Source: John Wiley & Sons, Inc.

FIGURE 17-2:
Image of an open and closed dome.

Open fit is a relatively new concept in hearing aids. It allows for more natural sound to enter your ear and prevents the occlusion effect — that is, when you perceive your own voice as a booming echo.

REMEMBER

Open fit is a great option to improve sound quality, but it's *only for those with mild, high-frequency hearing losses*. Closed domes address moderate and severe degrees of hearing loss and can add a boost to volume when needed. Hearing loss can range in degree from mild to profound and does not occur uniformly across frequencies (pitches). For most people, hearing loss occurs in the higher frequencies while leaving the lower frequencies normal or near-normal (see Chapters 3 and 7 for more on this). Be sure to consult a professional or the packaging to make sure a device's open fit options will work for your level of hearing loss.

We review several technical details of the many types and styles of hearing aids in deeper detail in Chapter 9.

Insuring Your Hearing Aids with a Trial Period Warranty

Traditionally, prescription hearing aids come with a state-mandated 45- to 60-day trial period during which you can return the hearing aids, and most manufacturers offer a standard two- to three-year warranty that includes general repairs and one-time replacement per hearing aid if it is lost or destroyed. Warranties for OTC hearing aids may vary considerably.

TIP

Particularly in the OTC hearing aid market, read the manufacturer's warranty closely. Specifically look for how long the warranty offers coverage, the kinds of damage covered, and the process for using the warranty. A robust warranty is a good sign that the manufacturer has faith in its product! A little research up front can help you make the right choice in the end.

TIP

Look for options to purchase warranty extensions or insurance if the initial warranty runs out for your hearing aids. These may be offered through the manufacturer or other private companies.

Customizing and Supporting Your Hearing Aids

This consideration is mostly aimed at OTC hearing aids. When selecting a prescription hearing aid, the hearing care professional is a vital part of the process and will customize the fit of your hearing aids with specialized equipment like real ear measures (see Chapter 9) and offer counseling and support.

REMEMBER

Remember that when using an OTC hearing aid, while it may be sold directly to you and not through a licensed hearing care professional, you can still see a hearing care professional to help with any adjustments needed.

Customizing any hearing aid output to your specific hearing can make a huge difference in your sound quality. If you're not working with a professional, you'll likely do one of the following to customize your OTC devices:

>> Select from a series of preconfigured profiles with a push button on the hearing aid or a remote control. These preconfigured profiles apply fixed volume settings across frequencies that are designed to address the most common patterns of hearing loss, but they are not truly customized.

>> Use a connected smartphone app to customize the output.

>> Work with a manufacturer's support team to set the device.

Make sure you do some research ahead of time into how an OTC device customizes the output and be sure it is a process you're comfortable with.

TIP

When purchasing OTC hearing aids, we recommend you look for smartphone apps that use some form of a hearing test to customize your hearing aids. The hearing test may vary but customizing the hearing aid this way is a sign that the company is truly trying to meet your unique hearing needs.

Monitoring Health with Hearing Aids

Hearing aids are constantly evolving and innovating. New hearing aids are inserting biosensors into the devices to monitor things like daily steps, falls, and heart rate.

In the future we may see more advanced and new health and wellness sensors integrated into hearing aids like information on changes in your overall physical activity and social activity levels, preemptive warnings on changes in balance or likelihood of experiencing a fall, changes in your body temperature, or daily cardiovascular monitoring beyond heart rate. There are a lot of possibilities, and it's super exciting to think of hearing aids as a central hub for health and wellness monitoring.

If you are the kind of person who likes feedback on your daily step count and keeping an eye on various health measures, consider looking for hearing aids that offer these features.

Accessorizing Your Hearing Aids

Many hearing aids have an array of complementary accessories and smartphone apps to help maximize the benefit by overcoming difficult situations or streamlining usage — just like some weather environments require a little something extra to make it through difficult situations. Imagine living in northern Alaska and not having snow tires. Hearing aids are no different; sometimes they require that something extra. Look for these add-ons when deciding on a hearing aid:

>> **Remote controls** allow you to change the hearing aid volume, settings, and programs without having to fiddle with tiny buttons on the hearing aid. Remote controls can be extremely useful when you have dexterity concerns or numbness in your fingers that makes finding and pressing buttons on the hearing aid difficult.

>> **Remote microphones** are wireless microphones that send a direct signal to the hearing aid anywhere from 30 to 90 feet away. These products are a fantastic way to overcome background noise issues or distance issues. Just place the remote microphone close to the speaker you want to hear, and you'll have a direct signal of their voice without as much background noise.

>> **TV connectors** plug into your television and send a direct sound signal to your hearing aids. With these connectors, you receive custom and clear audio signals from your television through your hearing aids for easy listening.

TIP

Look for OTC hearing aids that offer accessories. Even if you don't plan to use some of them right away, it is a sign of a company investing the time and effort to build a selection of hearing care products to meet various needs. Nearly all prescription hearing aids offer accessories.

Setting Expectations and Practicing

We couldn't do it — we couldn't present a chapter on considerations for hearing aid purchases without mentioning the most important considerations when using a hearing aid: setting realistic expectations for your hearing aids and practicing wearing them. This will take you further toward meeting your hearing goals than the hearing aids themselves, no matter the style, brand, or features.

We want you to start your journey knowing that hearing aids are not a cure for hearing loss and can't restore your hearing to normal. Many people fail to benefit from their hearing aids and stop using them because their expectations do not align with reality. While hearing aids may not correct hearing loss, they can still help you achieve your hearing goals and significantly improve your life, including your physical, emotional, and cognitive health. They do this by using many features and sound processing techniques to make sound work for you.

But it takes time and effort to adjust to new hearing aids. This is where practice makes perfect. Wear your hearing aids as often as possible and be mindful of what you're hearing. Put yourself in difficult listening situations purposefully to learn to use your hearing aids. Your patterns of hearing aid use may change over time as your find out what works best for you but early on, it's helpful to set aside dedicated extra time to practice. See Chapter 11 for some tips.

Chapter **18**

Ten Everyday Strategies to Hear Better

Hearing well means communicating well. And communication is what we do, all day, every day, with the people around us whom we care about and interact with.

It's easy to forget how foundational hearing is to everything we do in our lives. The everyday communication strategies in this chapter can make communicating with others and engaging with the world just a bit easier.

Get Close and Face-to-Face

Ideally, be at arm's length with the person you want to talk to. Sound loudness and quality both drop off quickly with increasing distance from the speaker. You want to be face-to-face with the person you're speaking with as well. For example, at a restaurant, it'll be easier for you to be across from the person you want to speak with rather than next to the person, despite your being close to the person in both situations. The visual cues of lip movements and facial expressions make it much easier for the brain to quickly translate sounds into meaning.

Recognize the Hearing Needs of the People You're Talking With

While you may struggle at times with hearing, you can be pretty darn sure that many other people you speak with are also likely dealing with the same problems as well. Having a sense of the hearing needs of others you're speaking with then is hugely important in knowing which strategies you can use to optimize communication, both for yourself and other people with whom you're speaking.

Be vigilant and look for non-verbal cues that can tell you if people are having trouble hearing you:

» They appear slightly puzzled (for example, eyebrow creasing) as they listen to you.

» They stare intently at your lips or face.

» Their non-verbal acknowledgments (a smile or nod of the head) of what you're saying is delayed.

Verbal cues are a bit more obvious:

» They pause intently before responding in the conversation.

» They frequently say they can't hear you or ask you to repeat yourself.

» They ask you repeatedly to stop mumbling when you're not.

It's okay to make some assumptions about someone's hearing based on their age. We all lose hearing as we age, and nearly two-thirds of everyone over 70 have meaningful hearing loss that can interfere with daily communication. So if you're talking to an older adult, it never hurts to go out of your way to follow some of the communication strategies summarized in this chapter and detailed more fully in Chapters 8 and 14.

Turn Down the Background Sounds

The sound quality of whatever you or others are trying to hear — whether it's a friend's voice or the dialog from a movie — will be much better if other sounds aren't competing with it. These other sounds can directly interfere with the voices you want to hear or make it much harder for your brain to distinguish the voice you're trying to hear. So, if you're having a conversation, for example, turn off the TV or radio, or move into a quieter part of the room.

Don't Just Ask "Huh?"

When you can't quite hear what someone said or you missed a word or two, rather than replying with a reflexive "Huh?" or "What?" it's far more helpful to quickly summarize what you did hear and ask for clarification.

For example, if your spouse is asking you about plans for the evening, but you only caught a few words around "dinner," you could ask, "What did you say about dinner?"

For the speaker, this makes it a lot easier since the speaker now knows exactly what to repeat. Importantly, it also shows the speaker that you were actually trying to listen (rather than purposely ignoring the speaker as many spouses complain is the case!).

Choose Good Listening Environments

Reverberation refers to the natural echoing of sounds when they bounce off walls and other surfaces. Reverberation interferes terribly when it comes to understanding speech. These echoes degrade the quality of speech sounds tremendously, making it much harder for everyone to hear each other. When picking out a room or restaurant to have a conversation in, look for rooms that have these qualities, which reduce reverberation:

>> Lower ceilings

>> Smaller rooms

>> Soft surfaces (such as rugs, drapes, pillows, upholstered furniture, and carpeted surfaces)

Also choose rooms with good lighting (no more dark corners of a restaurant!) so listeners have easy access to the visual cues of other people's faces and lips.

Use Closed Captioning

Captions (also known as subtitles) on TV are required by federal policy in the United States and are generally available with both live TV (such as news shows and sporting events) and prerecorded movies and shows. This feature is built into nearly all televisions and is also available on digital streaming services such as

Amazon, AppleTV, Disney Plus, HBO Max, Hulu, and Netflix. You can also find captions on video chat programs such as Cisco Webex, Google Meet, Microsoft Teams, Skype, and Zoom. Turning on captions makes it far easier for your brain to interpret sounds and can make watching movies and shows easier for everyone.

Wear Headphones When Listening to Music or Watching Media

Using headphones when listening to music or watching shows or movies on a TV or device can dramatically improve sound quality and make it much easier to understand the dialog and reduce the effort of listening. That's because headphones, particularly better quality headphones that completely cover your ears (as opposed to earbuds), deliver a clearer sound straight to your ears.

In most instances when you're listening to music or watching TV, the speaker is far enough from you that the sounds can become distorted by the time they reach your ears. Often, TV and devices also have poor internal speakers, reducing the sound quality.

TIP

On a smartphone or laptop, you just plug the headphones into the headphone jack or set up a Bluetooth connection. For TV, you can purchase various options for sending sound wirelessly from the output jack of your TV straight to a pair of headphones. The options available depend on the type of TV you have and the connections available on the TV.

Use Video Calls or VOIP When Calling Others

Phone calls made over VOIP (voice over internet protocol) services, such as FaceTime, Google Voice, Skype, and WhatsApp, all typically have wideband audio. This means that the frequency range of sounds being transmitted on the phone call can extend from 50 to 7,000 Hz, which makes the sound quality *so* much better than regular phone calls. You'll notice when making a call on any of these services that voices will sound more full or lifelike. This improved sound quality can make a huge difference with speech understanding, particularly if you have some underlying hearing loss.

An added benefit of many of the VOIP services, such as FaceTime, Skype, What'sApp, and Zoom, is that they allow for video calls as well. Having both the video component (with visual and lip cues) and audio signal can make it a lot easier for you to understand speech.

Customize the Hearing and Sound Features on Your Smartphone

Seriously, what did we do before we had those mini-computers in our pockets all day? Smartphones can do millions of things. But did you know smartphones can customize sound to your needs and even act as handheld amplifiers?

Apps on smartphones can test your hearing and use those tests to customize the sound to your specific hearing levels. This can improve ease of listening and sound quality. In addition, you can use the smartphone to amplify sounds around you when needed. For example, in a noisy restaurant, you can place the smartphone on the table and use an amplifier app for a boost in hearing others at the table. Some apps even have background noise reduction programs. Check out your Apple or Android app store for options which, at time of publication of this book, include apps such as Chatable, Google Sound Amplifier, Mimi, and Sonic Cloud.

Know Your Hearing Number

Knowledge is power. And better yet, precise knowledge is even more powerful. To understand your own hearing needs and those of others, get familiar with your hearing number (also known clinically as the pure-tone average). This number reflects how loud speech sounds have to be for you to hear them and can be directly calculated from an audiogram or any number of smartphone apps (see Chapter 7). Knowing your hearing number and possibly that of other close family members allows you to understand your and others' hearing needs and what communication strategies are needed to optimize your hearing.

Chapter **19**

Ten Myths about Hearing Loss

As clinicians, we're used to hearing all sorts of wacky stuff about hearing, which often stems from the public not having access to clear, easily accessible information on hearing loss. This is in many ways why we chose to write this book. Read on for some of the most common myths we've encountered when talking to our patients and in the broader media.

Hearing Loss Is Just Part of Getting Older so It Can't Be That Important

Sigh . . . there's a tendency to dump hearing loss into the same category as graying hair and wrinkles: an inevitable and innocuous process that comes with aging. In contrast, we make high blood pressure — another condition that often comes with aging — a priority, understanding the impact that it can have on strokes and heart attacks.

Over the past ten years, researchers have come to understand that hearing loss has objective and significant effects on our health and well-being, including our social relationships, risk of falls, depression, and risk of cognitive decline and dementia. Hearing and communicating have an impact on everything we do on a daily basis. Most importantly, clinicians and researchers believe that addressing hearing loss through the communication strategies and technologies we discuss in this book can make a difference in helping keep us engaged and healthy.

My Hearing Is Fine; It's Just That Everyone Is Mumbling

Ha! Speech that comes across as mumbling is exactly what hearing loss sounds like. Hearing loss develops as the inner ear (*cochlea*) ages and can no longer send clear signals to the brain. To our brains, this sounds exactly as if people are mumbling all the time. Some situations are better (or worse) than others. Talking in a quiet room with someone sitting close and face-to-face with you, you'll notice far fewer issues with your hearing loss than in settings with background noise or a speaker who is far away.

Trouble Hearing? Just Have People Shout!

People shouting does not fix what you can't hear! And it can actually be harmful. Most hearing loss is a clarity issue, not a volume issue. This is because hearing loss doesn't affect all parts of sound equally. We experience hearing loss at different frequencies, or pitches. Most people have trouble with high-pitched sounds. So just making everything louder by shouting doesn't help. In fact, it can make things worse because shouting distorts sound. Instead, people with hearing loss need targeted amplification to meet their hearing needs. Rather than asking people to talk louder, ask them to speak slowly at a slightly louder than normal level, and make sure you can see their mouths to help with lip reading (which we all do, consciously or subconsciously).

I'll Wait to Get My Hearing Tested Until I Notice a Problem

You may not even realize that you have a hearing loss until you get your hearing tested. The very nature of how we hear makes noticing hearing loss very difficult. First, hearing loss occurs slowly over time — so slowly, in fact, that our brains constantly adjust to our surroundings and barely notice a change. Second, our brains are bombarded with sounds all day long and do a great job of learning what to ignore or pay attention to. This means we're actually preprogrammed to ignore sounds that aren't interesting to us. But sound is invisible and can't be felt to the touch, so we have no way to know what we're missing.

People are notoriously bad at judging their own hearing. Instead of taking a wait-and-see approach, be proactive. Get your hearing testing professionally or use a self-testing app on a smartphone to learn your hearing number and monitor it over time (see Chapter 7). Then continue to check your hearing every year or so. If you don't have hearing loss now, you'll have a baseline. If you do, rest assured that taking action on your part — such as using hearing aids earlier rather than later — can help make the adjustment process easier.

I'll Address My Hearing Loss Later When It Gets Really Bad

Waiting until your hearing gets really bad is not a good way to approach hearing loss. Procrastination in general is not a good thing and particularly with any type of health issue. You certainly wouldn't want to ignore your high blood pressure until you have a stroke or your arthritis until you can no longer easily walk. Nearly any health issue is best addressed earlier rather than later. The same goes for hearing loss. The longer your hearing loss goes unaddressed, the more detrimental its potential effects on the quality of your relationships and on your cognitive and brain health. Likewise, the longer the brain goes without access to sound, the harder it'll be later for your brain to get used to and learn how to use the sounds from a hearing aid. As we hope we convey in this book, though, treating your hearing loss doesn't necessarily mean you run out and buy hearing aids at the first sign of hearing loss.

I Have Hearing Loss. Now I Need Hearing Aids?

The overwhelming belief is that having any hearing loss means needing hearing aids. But it's so much more nuanced than that. No two people experience hearing loss the exact same way — some with a mild hearing loss are able to compensate with ease while others with the same mild hearing loss are completely unable to adjust and begin to withdraw from social activities. The point at which someone requires hearing aids varies.

Hearing care is meant to consist of a toolkit of options to meet your hearing needs. While hearing aids are the most common way to address hearing loss, they are just one item in the toolkit. Other options include:

» Simple environmental modifications like seeking good lighting or avoiding background noise

» Letting other people know how they can help you hear better, such as coming closer or refraining from putting their hands in front of their mouths

» Communication tips (such as getting face-to-face when talking; see Chapter 8)

» Use of a smartphone speech-to-text app in noisy settings

» Personal amplifiers (PSAPs) for difficult situations

» Cochlear implants

Hearing Aids Fix Your Hearing

Ahhhhhh (that's the sound of Frank and Nick screaming)!!!! The idea that hearing aids "fix" hearing loss is clearly the biggest myth of all, and it's perpetuated by all the marketing you see about hearing aids. Hearing aids don't fix your hearing problems any more than a prosthetic leg "fixes" the challenges of having a lower leg amputation. A hearing aid certainly helps with hearing and communication, but it also needs to be coupled with using communication strategies and optimizing external factors that can improve the sound quality of what you're trying to hear (see Chapter 8). With hearing loss, the inner ear is damaged, so a range of technologies and strategies are needed to help the brain understand the sounds coming from the ear.

I Can Just Put in My Hearing Aids and They'll Work Fine

Even people who accept that hearing aids don't return hearing to normal may still expect to simply put hearing aids in their ears and go about their business from day one. Don't be fooled into this mindset by overzealous advertising.

Hearing aids are amazing devices, but using hearing aids takes effort on your part! You need to put in the time to practice using them in various listening situations and take a mindful approach to adjusting to the new sound of your hearing aids. This advice is not meant to discourage you. On the contrary, we want you to go in with the right mindset to ensure your success!

A Cochlear Implant Is Only for People Who Are Completely Deaf

The idea that only people who are totally deaf can benefit from a cochlear implant is a huge myth! The vast majority of those who get cochlear implants are now adults in their 70s, 80s, and even 90s who have progressively lost hearing over time and are finding that they're still struggling to communicate, even with hearing aids. When in a quiet room with a single speaker, these patients can often still communicate okay, but in other situations, they will struggle. If you've been told that you have a moderate hearing loss or worse (or your hearing number is in the 60s or higher) and you're struggling to communicate with hearing aids in any place other than a quiet room with a single speaker, we recommend that you be evaluated for a cochlear implant or at least find out more. Nearly all academic centers and larger private ear, nose, and throat (ENT) practices have a cochlear implant program where you can get evaluated. The evaluation and cochlear implants are routinely covered by health insurance.

I Should Keep My Hearing Loss to Myself

No. Just don't. Don't make your hearing loss a secret. There is nothing embarrassing about hearing loss. The environment around you and the people you interact with play a big role in hearing and communication. Even with hearing aids or cochlear implants, you can only do so much to address your hearing, and you'll still encounter difficult situations such as background noise.

Sometimes seeking changes and accommodations in situations can help you hear and communicate better (see Chapter 8). Unfortunately, people don't know you or your hearing needs. Rather than keeping it to yourself in isolation, speak up! Let people know what kinds of communication styles work best for you or if you'd like to move away from a noise source that is making it hard for you to hear.

Communication, by nature, involves multiple participants. When we're open about hearing loss, everyone can benefit from knowing how to participate.

Index

earmuffs, protective, 38–39

earphones, 9–10, 39–40, 242

earplugs, 38–39

earwax, 43–44, 162–163, 165

eczema, 44

electronic dryers, 161

emergency hearing tests, 69–70

ENT physician. *See* ear, nose, and throat physician

estrogen, 9, 36

Eustachian tube, 24, 26, 30, 42

expectations, realistic
  for cochlear implants, 191–192
  for hearing aids, 142, 151–153, 237, 248–249

external ear
  conductive hearing loss, 30
  infections in, 24, 30, 41, 187–188
  overview, 23, 24

eyeglasses, 200

F

FaceTime, 117, 203, 242–243

face-to-face communication, 111, 201, 239

facial expressions, 111

fall risk due to hearing loss, 11, 56

FDA (U.S. Food and Drug Administration), 144–145, 234

feedback, avoiding, 128, 158, 165

feedback suppression feature, 140

fitting hearing aids, 141–142

Flexible Spending Account, paying for hearing aids with, 216

fluid in middle ear, 42, 188

FM systems, 180–181

follow-up appointments after hearing aid purchase, 142

Food and Drug Administration (FDA), U.S., 144–145, 234

foreign objects in ear, 30

free hearing tests, 76, 208

frequency lowering feature, 141

frequency of sound, 20–21, 93, 125–126

G

gender, as risk factor, 9, 36

genetics, effect on hearing loss, 36–37

Google Voice, 117, 203, 242–243

gradual hearing loss, 64, 246–247

group setting remote microphones, 175, 176

H

HAC (hearing aid compatible) technology, 180

headphones, 9–10, 39–40, 242

health
  impact of hearing loss on, 10–11
  monitoring with hearing aids, 236

Health Savings Account, paying for hearing aids with, 216

hearing, process of
  decoding of sound by brain, 8, 26–29, 31, 110
  ear anatomy, 23–26
  understanding sound, 20–23

hearing aid accessories. *See* accessories, hearing aid

Hearing Aid Compatibility Act, 180

hearing aid compatible (HAC) technology, 180

hearing aids. *See also* cost of hearing aids; over-the-counter hearing aids; prescription hearing aids; purchasing hearing aids; styles of hearing aids
  adaptation process, 69, 153–156
  adjusting, 159–160
  advanced signal processing techniques, 127
  basic versus premium, 149–150
  batteries, 157
  Bluetooth and, 171–172
  bundling of hearing care services, 209–210, 215
  clarity of sound, enhancing with, 126–128
  cleaning of, 162–163
  compression, 125
  dementia, preventing with, 59
  determining need for, 104–105, 247–248
  directionality feature, 127, 140, 149
  dryers for, 161
  features of, 140–141

sound quality, 29, 32, 110

SoundPrint app, 115

speaking up about hearing loss, 117–120, 249

specialized tests of sound processing, 89

spectrograms, 21–23

speech awareness threshold, 87

speech enhancement feature, 140

speech in noise tests, 87–88

speech reception testing, 86–87

speech reception threshold, 86, 100

speech understanding, measuring, 86–88

speech-frequency pure-tone average, 13

SSA benefits. *See* Social Security Administration benefits

SSD (single-sided deafness), 16, 137–138, 191, 192–194

SSDI (Social Security Disability Insurance), 222

SSI (Supplemental Security Income), 222

SSNHL (sudden sensorineural hearing loss), 43, 186

stapes, 25

steroids, 186

stiffening of ear bones, 188

stigma of hearing loss, overcoming, 70–73

storage of hearing aids, 160–161

stores, purchasing OTC hearing aids at, 146

streamers, 172, 177

styles of hearing aids

  behind-the-ear, 128–132

  choosing, 230–232

  in-the-ear, 132–133

  open and closed styles, 131–132

  overview, 128

  pros and cons of, 133–134

  receiver-in-the-canal BTE, 131

  slim tube BTE, 130

  traditional BTE, 129–130

substantial gainful activity, 224

subtitles. *See* captioning

sudden sensorineural hearing loss (SSNHL), 43, 186

summarizing and repeating strategy, 111–112, 241

Supplemental Security Income (SSI), 222

support for people with hearing loss, 17, 204–205

support groups, 120–121

surgeries

  cochlear implants, 189–192

  for conductive hearing loss, 188–189

  evaluation, paying for, 208

  implantable hearing devices, 192–194

  overview, 188

  for sensorineural hearing loss, 189–192

swimmer's ear, 41

T

T rating, 180

table remote microphones, 175, 176

Technical Stuff icon, 3

technology, hearing assistive. *See* hearing assistive technology

technology strategies, 115–117, 202–203

telecoil

  versus Bluetooth, 181–182

  FM systems, 180–181

  infrared systems, 181

  overview, 178

  public hearing loop systems, 178–179

  purchasing hearing aids with, 233

  telephones and, 180

telephones. *See also* smartphones

  ADA requirements for, 221

  captioned, 168–169

  telecoil and, 180

  VOIP calls, 116–117, 203, 242–243

temporal lobe, 26–27

third-party disability, 53

tinnitus, 46–48

Tip icon, 3

traditional BTE, 129–130, 134

About the Authors

Frank R. Lin, MD, PhD, is Professor of Otolaryngology and Epidemiology and the Director of the Cochlear Center for Hearing and Public Health at Johns Hopkins University. As an otologic surgeon and epidemiologist, Dr. Lin has translated his clinical experiences caring for patients with hearing loss into foundational public health research and federal policy in the United States. His research established the association of hearing loss with cognitive decline and dementia, and he now leads an ongoing, National Institutes of Health-funded randomized trial investigating into whether hearing loss treatment can reduce the risk of cognitive decline and dementia in older adults. In parallel, Dr. Lin has collaborated with the National Academies, White House, and Congress to develop policies to ensure hearing loss can be effectively and sustainably addressed in society. These efforts directly resulted in bipartisan passage of the Over-the-Counter Hearing Aid Act of 2017, which Dr. Lin testified on before Congress. In addition to his work, he spends most days in his hometown of Baltimore, Maryland, with his wife and family, shuttling his three kids between school and other activities and trying to find time for a run. Unlike his young'un coauthor, Nick Reed, he actually remembers the Baltimore Orioles winning a World Series way back in '83 and is equally hopeful that he'll see another one while his kids are still kids.

Nicholas S. Reed, AuD, is Assistant Professor in the Department of Epidemiology at Johns Hopkins Bloomberg School of Public Health with a joint appointment as an audiologist in the Department of Otolaryngology-Head and Neck Surgery at Johns Hopkins School of Medicine. He completed his audiology degree at Towson University in Maryland and his clinical training at Georgetown University Hospital. During his training, he became concerned with the lack of access and affordability to hearing care in the United States and considered leaving audiology all together. After meeting his longtime mentor and coauthor, Frank Lin, he rededicated his life to research and policy initiatives to improve hearing care for the millions of people with hearing loss around the world. His work focuses on direct-to-consumer hearing care solutions, hearing care policy in the United States, integrating hearing measures into epidemiologic studies across the globe, and building sustainable solutions for a healthcare system to accommodate the needs of people with hearing loss to improve patient-provider communication, satisfaction with care, and long-term health outcomes. His work has been featured in major media outlets including *CBS Sunday Morning* and the *New York Times*. On any given day, he can be found in his hometown, Baltimore, Maryland, thinking about hearing loss, begging his Nonna to make any of her native Sicilian dishes for family dinner, wondering if he'll ever see a world series title from his beloved Baltimore Orioles in his lifetime, and hanging out with his wife and sons.

Dedication

My earliest memories involve my grandmother, now 99 years old, who helped raise me and has long struggled with her hearing loss. She and my parents, who are both public health physicians and researchers, inspired me on my current path and made this book possible. A special thanks also goes out to my wife (Helen) and kids (Audrey, Nate, and Connor) for always being supportive and for making life fun.

—Frank Lin

This book is dedicated to every single patient I've ever had the pleasure of serving. I have learned more from you than through any text or course. Thank you for trusting me and teaching me. It's also dedicated to my family, who instilled a commitment to others from an early age and push me every day to be better. Thank you to my mom, dad, grandparents, brother, and especially my wife, Katie, and my sons, Sammy and baby boy Reed (due October 2022) — thanks for letting me skip all the *Winnie the Pooh* or *Toy Story* movie night viewings to work on this book instead.

—Nicholas Reed

Authors' Acknowledgments

Special thanks to the people at AARP — especially Jodi Lipson and Charlotte Yeh, who provided continuous feedback and review as we developed this book. Every chapter in this book was improved by their knowledge, insights, and experience.

We also want to thank all the amazing people at John Wiley & Sons, Inc. Special recognition goes to Tracy Boggier, Kristie Pyles, and Christy Pingleton. A huge shout-out goes particularly to Linda Brandon who put up with our constant questioning on how best to frame various concepts in this book and her invaluable edits that greatly improved this book.

Publisher's Acknowledgments

Senior Acquisitions Editor: Tracy Boggier
Development Editor: Linda Brandon
Copy Editor: Christy Pingleton
Proofreader: Debbye Butler

Production Editor: Mohammed Zafar Ali
Cover Image: © peterschreiber.media/ Shutterstock

Take dummies with you everywhere you go!

Whether you are excited about e-books, want more from the web, must have your mobile apps, or are swept up in social media, dummies makes everything easier.

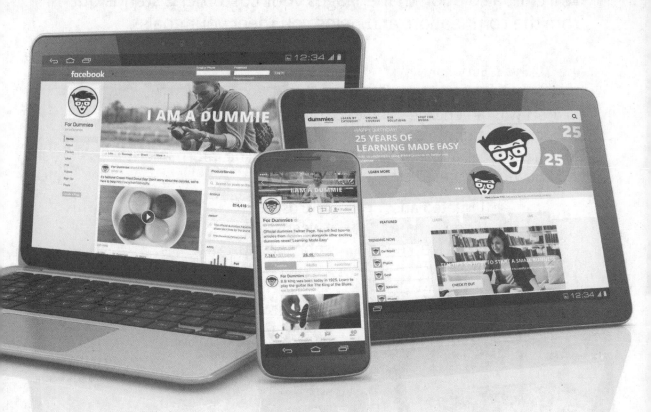

Find us online!

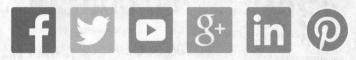

dummies.com

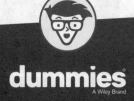

dummies
A Wiley Brand

Leverage the power

Dummies is the global leader in the reference category and one of the most trusted and highly regarded brands in the world. No longer just focused on books, customers now have access to the dummies content they need in the format they want. Together we'll craft a solution that engages your customers, stands out from the competition, and helps you meet your goals.

Advertising & Sponsorships

Connect with an engaged audience on a powerful multimedia site, and position your message alongside expert how-to content. Dummies.com is a one-stop shop for free, online information and know-how curated by a team of experts.

- Targeted ads
- Video
- Email Marketing
- Microsites
- Sweepstakes sponsorship

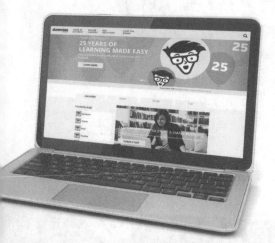

20 MILLION PAGE VIEWS EVERY SINGLE MONTH

15 MILLION UNIQUE VISITORS PER MONTH

43% OF ALL VISITORS ACCESS THE SITE VIA THEIR MOBILE DEVICES

700,000 NEWSLETTER SUBSCRIPTIONS TO THE INBOXES OF

300,000 UNIQUE INDIVIDUALS EVERY WEEK

# of dummies

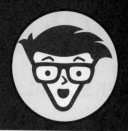

Custom Publishing

Reach a global audience in any language by creating a solution that will differentiate you from competitors, amplify your message, and encourage customers to make a buying decision.

- Apps
- Books
- eBooks
- Video
- Audio
- Webinars

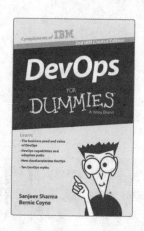
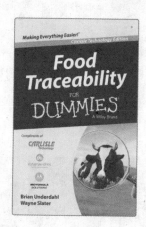
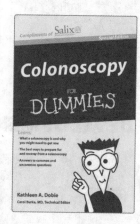
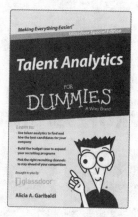

Brand Licensing & Content

Leverage the strength of the world's most popular reference brand to reach new audiences and channels of distribution.

For more information, visit **dummies.com/biz**

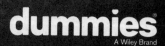

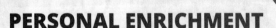

PERSONAL ENRICHMENT

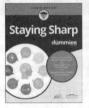

Staying Sharp dummies

9781119187790
USA $26.00
CAN $31.99
UK £19.99

Facebook dummies
Carolyn Abram

9781119179030
USA $21.99
CAN $25.99
UK £16.99

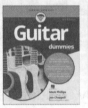

Guitar dummies
Mark Phillips
Jon Chappell

9781119293354
USA $24.99
CAN $29.99
UK £17.99

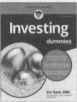

Investing dummies
Eric Tyson, MBA

9781119293347
USA $22.99
CAN $27.99
UK £16.99

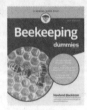

Beekeeping dummies
Howland Blackiston

9781119310068
USA $22.99
CAN $27.99
UK £16.99

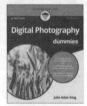

Digital Photography dummies
Julie Adair King

9781119235606
USA $24.99
CAN $29.99
UK £17.99

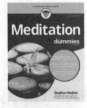

Meditation dummies
Stephan Bodian

9781119251163
USA $24.99
CAN $29.99
UK £17.99

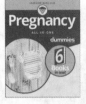

Pregnancy ALL-IN-ONE dummies
6 Books in one

9781119235491
USA $26.99
CAN $31.99
UK £19.99

Samsung Galaxy S7 dummies
Bill Hughes

9781119279952
USA $24.99
CAN $29.99
UK £17.99

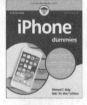

iPhone dummies
Edward C. Baig
Bob "Dr. Mac" LeVitus

9781119283133
USA $24.99
CAN $29.99
UK £17.99

Crocheting dummies
Karen Manthey
Susan Brittain

9781119287117
USA $24.99
CAN $29.99
UK £16.99

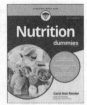

Nutrition dummies
Carol Ann Rinzler

9781119130246
USA $22.99
CAN $27.99
UK £16.99

PROFESSIONAL DEVELOPMENT

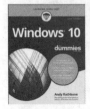

Windows 10 dummies
Andy Rathbone

9781119311041
USA $24.99
CAN $29.99
UK £17.99

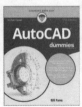

AutoCAD dummies
Bill Fane

9781119255796
USA $39.99
CAN $47.99
UK £27.99

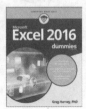

Excel 2016 dummies
Greg Harvey, PhD

9781119293439
USA $26.99
CAN $31.99
UK £19.99

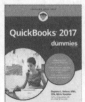

QuickBooks 2017 dummies
Stephen L. Nelson, MBA, CPA, MS in Taxation

9781119281467
USA $26.99
CAN $31.99
UK £19.99

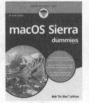

macOS Sierra dummies
Bob "Dr. Mac" LeVitus

9781119280651
USA $29.99
CAN $35.99
UK £21.99

LinkedIn dummies
Joel Elad, MBAs

9781119251132
USA $24.99
CAN $29.99
UK £17.99

Windows 10 ALL-IN-ONE dummies
10 Books in one
Woody Leonhard

9781119310563
USA $34.00
CAN $41.99
UK £24.99

SharePoint 2016 dummies
Rosemarie Withee
Ken Withee

9781119181705
USA $29.99
CAN $35.99
UK £21.99

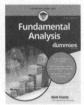

Fundamental Analysis dummies
Matt Krantz

9781119263593
USA $26.99
CAN $31.99
UK £19.99

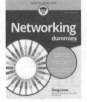

Networking dummies
Doug Lowe

9781119257769
USA $29.99
CAN $35.99
UK £21.99

Office 2016 dummies
Wallace Wang

9781119293477
USA $26.99
CAN $31.99
UK £19.99

Office 365 dummies
Rosemarie Withee
Ken Withee
Jennifer Reed

9781119265313
USA $24.99
CAN $29.99
UK £17.99

Salesforce.com dummies
Liz Kao
Jon Paz

9781119239314
USA $29.99
CAN $35.99
UK £21.99

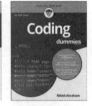

Coding dummies
Nikhil Abraham

9781119293323
USA $29.99
CAN $35.99
UK £21.99

dummies.com

dummies A Wiley Brand

Learning Made Easy

ACADEMIC

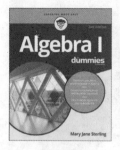

9781119293576
USA $19.99
CAN $23.99
UK £15.99

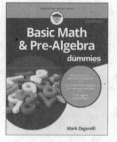

9781119293637
USA $19.99
CAN $23.99
UK £15.99

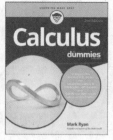

9781119293491
USA $19.99
CAN $23.99
UK £15.99

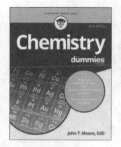

9781119293460
USA $19.99
CAN $23.99
UK £15.99

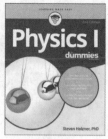

9781119293590
USA $19.99
CAN $23.99
UK £15.99

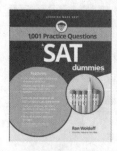

9781119215844
USA $26.99
CAN $31.99
UK £19.99

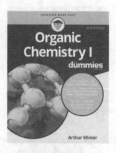

9781119293378
USA $22.99
CAN $27.99
UK £16.99

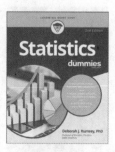

9781119293521
USA $19.99
CAN $23.99
UK £15.99

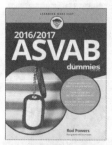

9781119239178
USA $18.99
CAN $22.99
UK £14.99

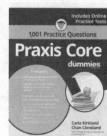

9781119263883
USA $26.99
CAN $31.99
UK £19.99

Available Everywhere Books Are Sold

dummies.com

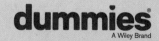
dummies®
A Wiley Brand

Small books for big imaginations

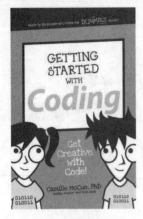

GETTING STARTED WITH Coding
Get Creative with Code!

Camille McCue, PhD

9781119177173
USA $9.99
CAN $9.99
UK £8.99

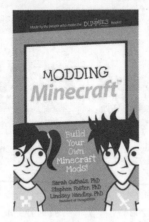

MODDING Minecraft™
Build Your Own Minecraft Mods!

Sarah Guthals, PhD
Stephen Foster, PhD
Lindsey Handley, PhD

9781119177272
USA $9.99
CAN $9.99
UK £8.99

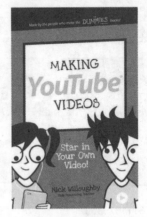

MAKING YouTube VIDEOS
Star in Your Own Video!

Nick Willoughby

9781119177241
USA $9.99
CAN $9.99
UK £8.99

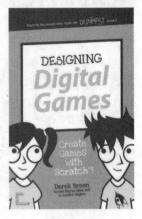

DESIGNING Digital Games
Create Games with Scratch™!

Derek Breen

9781119177210
USA $9.99
CAN $9.99
UK £8.99

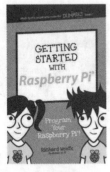

GETTING STARTED WITH Raspberry Pi®
Program Your Raspberry Pi®!

Richard Wentk

9781119262657
USA $9.99
CAN $9.99
UK £6.99

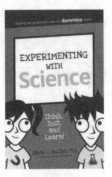

EXPERIMENTING WITH Science
Think, Test, and Learn!

Olivia J. Mullins, PhD

9781119291336
USA $9.99
CAN $9.99
UK £6.99

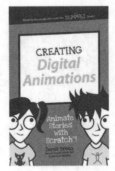

CREATING Digital Animations
Animate Stories with Scratch™!

Derek Breen

9781119233527
USA $9.99
CAN $9.99
UK £6.99

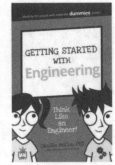

GETTING STARTED WITH Engineering
Think Like an Engineer!

Camille McCue, PhD

9781119291220
USA $9.99
CAN $9.99
UK £6.99

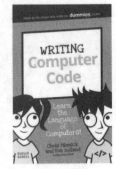

WRITING Computer Code
Learn the Language of Computers!

Chris Minnick and Eva Holland

9781119177302
USA $9.99
CAN $9.99
UK £8.99

Unleash Their Creativity

dummies.com

dummies®
A Wiley Brand